Mariam Kazim Jassab
Ali Aboulkadhim Aboulmahdi

Pesticides and Hard Ticks

Mariam Kazim Jassab
Ali Aboulkadhim Aboulmahdi

Pesticides and Hard Ticks

Noor Publishing

Imprint

Cover image: www.ingimage.com

Publisher:
Noor Publishing
is a trademark of
Dodo Books Indian Ocean Ltd. and OmniScriptum S.R.L publishing group

120 High Road, East Finchley, London, N2 9ED, United Kingdom
Str. Armeneasca 28/1, office 1, Chisinau MD-2012, Republic of Moldova, Europe
Managing Directors: Ieva Konstantinova, Victoria Ursu
info@omniscriptum.com

Printed at: see last page
ISBN: 978-620-9-50403-7

Pesticides and Hard Ticks

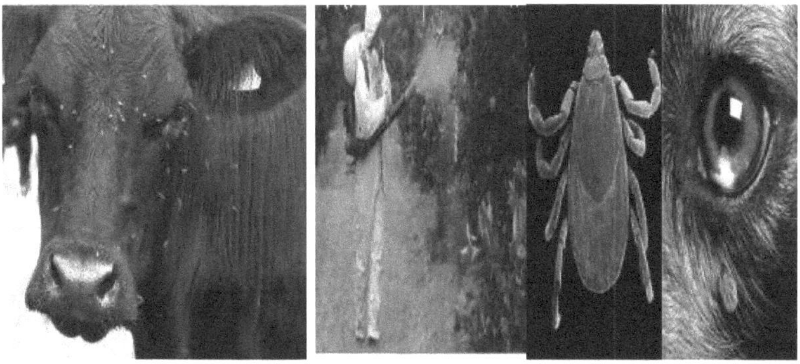

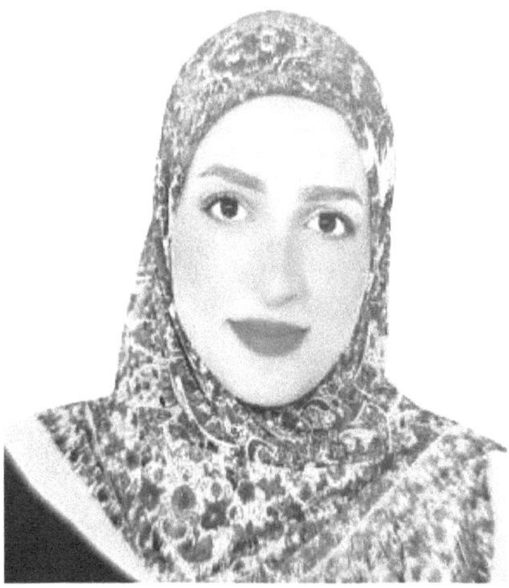

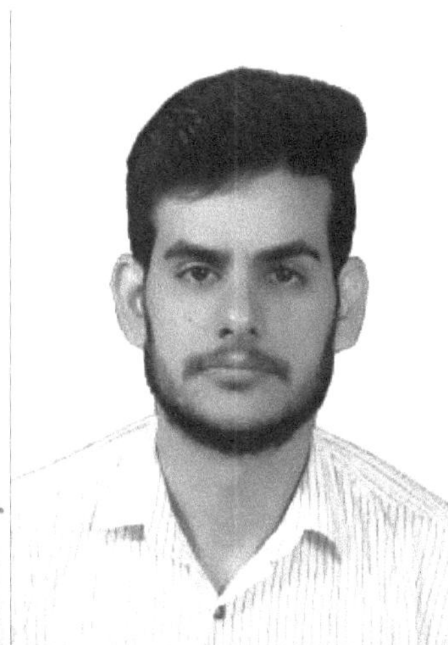

By

Dr. Mariam Kazim Jassab

Dr. ALI ABOULKADHIM ABOULMAHDI

(2026)

Pesticides and Hard Ticks

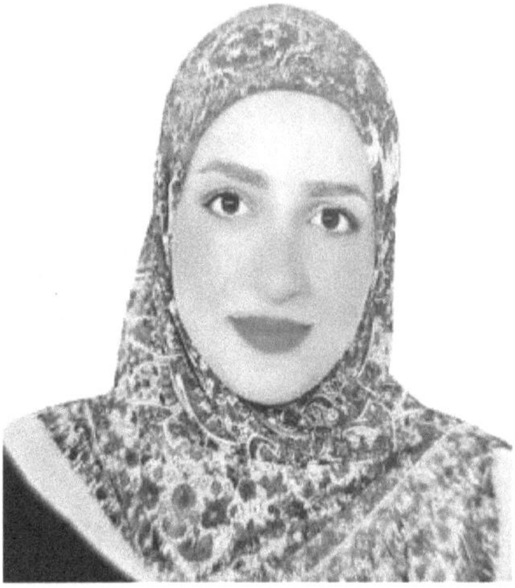

Dr. Mariam Kazim Jassab

Internal and Preventive Medicine

College of Veterinary Medicine Al-Qasim Green University, Iraq

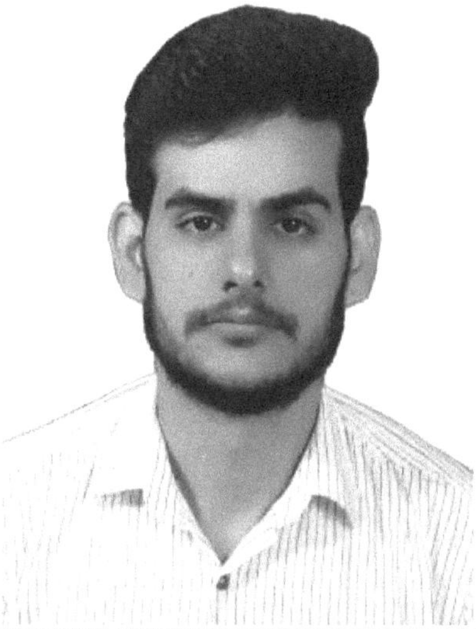

Dr. ALI ABOULKADHIM ABOULMAHDI

Babylon Veterinary Teaching Hospital, Iraq

Contents list

INTRODUCTION

Ticks are able to transmit tick-borne infectious agents to vertebrate hosts which cause major constraints to public and livestock health. The costs associated with mortality, relapse, treatments, and decreased production yields are economically significant.

Ticks adapted to a hematophagous existence after the vertebrate hemostatic system evolved into a multi-layered defense system against foreign invasion (pathogens and ectoparasites), blood loss, and immune responses. Subsequently, ticks evolved by developing an ability to suppress the vertebrate host immune system with a devastating impact particularly for exotic and crossbred cattle.

Host genetics defines the immune responsiveness against ticks and tick-borne pathogens. To gain an insight into the naturally acquired resistant and susceptible cattle breed against ticks, studies have been conducted comparing the incidence of tick infestation on bovine hosts from divergent genetic backgrounds.

It is well-documented that purebred and crossbred *Bos taurus indicus* cattle are more resistant to ticks and tick-borne pathogens compared to purebred European *Bos taurus taurus* cattle. Genetic studies identifying Quantitative Trait Loci markers using microsatellites and SNPs have been inconsistent with very low percentages relating phenotypic variation with tick infestation.

Several skin gene expression and immunological studies have been undertaken using different breeds, different samples (peripheral blood, skin with tick feeding), infestation protocols and geographic environments. Susceptible breeds were commonly found to be associated with the increased expression of toll like receptors, MHC Class II, calcium binding proteins, and complement factors with an increased presence of neutrophils in the skin following tick feeding.

Resistant breeds had higher levels of T cells present in the skin prior to tick infestation and thus seem to respond to ticks more efficiently. The skin of resistant breeds also contained higher numbers of eosinophils, mast cells and basophils with up-regulated proteases, cathepsins, keratins, collagens and extracellular matrix proteins in response to feeding ticks.

Vector-borne pathogens cause diseases with a great impact on public and veterinary health and have accounted for 22% of emerging infections between 1940 and 2004 (Jones et al., 2008). As obligate hematophagous arthropod pests of vertebrates, ticks pose serious threats to beef and dairy cattle producers.

It has been estimated that 80% of the world's cattle population is at risk from tick and tick-borne diseases (TBDs) causing estimated annual losses of US$ 22–30 billion (Lew-Tabor and Rodriguez Valle, 2016).

The negative impact of ticks on cattle production is due to the direct effects of feeding, such as weight loss and damage of leather, and indirect effects, such as the transmission of tick-borne pathogens. The resulting diseases can potentially cause major production losses in livestock, thereby reducing farm incomes, increasing costs to consumers, and threatening trade between regions and/or world markets.

Since the establishment of extensive vector control programs, a steady decline in vector-borne diseases was observed last century, however recently the emergence and re-emergence of vector-borne diseases has been observed.

This re-emergence may be linked to new global trends associated with changes in animal husbandry, urbanization, animal transboundary transportation, and globalization (Ogden and Lindsay, 2016). In this scenario, various approaches for tick control are in practice around the world in accordance with local legislation, environmental conditions, price based selection, and geography.

Acaricide (synthetic pesticides) application is the most common component of tick control strategies, however the use of acaricides impose numerous limitations including the selective pressure for the development of more resistant ticks, environmental contamination, drug residues in food products, the expense of developing new acaricides, and the difficulty of producing tick-resistant cattle while maintaining desirable production characteristics (Willadsen, 2004; Abbas et al., 2014).

Anti-tick vaccines are a very promising alternative to acaricide usage, however are still insufficient to confer protection against multiple tick species in various geographical regions (de la Fuente and Contreras, 2015; de la Fuente et al., 2016; Schetters et al., 2016).

Anti-tick immunity has been described in guinea pigs, cattle and rabbits, and refers to the capacity of previously exposed hosts to interfere with tick feeding and reproductive fecundity (Nuttall, 1911; Trager, 1939; Hewetson, 1972).

A reduction in tick weight, duration of attachment, number of ticks feeding, egg mass, and molting success are some of the parameters measured to determine host anti-tick immunity (Trager, 1939). For the first time, Nuttall (1911) demonstrated host immunity to ticks as a phenomenon of natural immunity in humans. Experimentally, acquired resistance to tick infestation was observed by Trager (1939), who noticed that after repeated infestation of *Dermacentor variabilis* on guinea pigs, the host developed resistance to subsequent tick infestation, shown by the decreasing number of successfully feeding larvae.

Furthermore, it was found that as compared with larvae infesting a host with no previous exposure to ticks, larvae infesting resistant hosts weighed less. Several researchers continued to observe host resistance to tick feeding affecting each tick life stage (Gregson, 1941; Feldman-Muhsam, 1964; Wikel, 1996).

Various immunological determinants have been examined that influence host resistance to tick infestation including a high level of eosinophils, basophils, T cells, mast cells, specific immunoglobulins, histamine, and changes to gene transcription profiles (Kemp and Bourne, 1980; de Castro and Newson, 1993; Kashino et al., 2005; Veríssimo et al., 2008; Kongsuwan et al., 2010; Piper et al., 2010; Engracia Filho et al., 2017).

Bovines present contrasting, heritable phenotypes for infestation with *Rhipicephalus microplus* and related tick species as a consequence of co-evolution of resistant cattle with ticks and also decades of selective breeding. The *R. microplus* tick has a strong preference for *Bos taurus taurus* cattle over highly resistant *Bos taurus indicus* cattle (Wambura et al., 1998; Porto Neto et al., 2011b; Jonsson et al., 2014; Biegelmeyer et al., 2015).

In this article we review the tick:host physical interface, genetic and molecular studies, and immunological determinants of bovine host resistance to ticks.

Parasitic diseases is a global problem and considered as a major obstacle in the health and product performance of animals. These may be due to endo-parasites that live inside the body or ecto-parasites such as ticks, mites, flies, fleas, midges, etc., which attack the body surface. Among ecto-parasites, ticks are very important and harmful blood sucking external parasites of mammals, birds and reptiles throughout the world (Furman and Loomis, 1984).

The medical and economic importance of ticks had long been recognized due to their ability to transmit diseases to humans and animals. Ticks belong to phylum, Arthropoda and make up the largest collection of creatures in order Acarina.

Ticks are divided into two groups: soft bodied ticks (Argasidae) and hard bodied species (Ixodidae).

Hard ticks feed for extended periods of time on their hosts, varying from several days to weeks, depending on such factors as life stage, host type, and species of tick.

The outside surface, or cuticle, of hard ticks actually grows to accommodate the large volume of blood ingested, which, in adult ticks, may be anywhere from 200 to 600 times their unfed body weight (Sonenshine, 1991).

Additionally, many soft ticks have an uncanny resistance to starvation, and can survive for many years without blood meal (Furman and Loomis, 1984).

The outside surface, or cuticle, of soft ticks expands, but does not grow to accommodate the large volume of blood ingested, which may be anywhere from 5 to 10 times their unfed body weight (Sonenshine, 1991).

Ticks cause great economic losses to livestock in the world and have adverse effect on livestock host in several ways (Snelson, 1975) and parasitize a wide range of vertebrate hosts, and transmit a wider variety of pathogenic agents than any other group of arthropods (Oliver, 1989).

There are 899 tick species those parasitize the vertebrates including Argasidae (185 species), Ixodidae (713 species) and Nuttalliellidae (1 specie) (Barker and Murrell, 2004).

Ticks are the most important ecto-parasites of livestock in tropical and sub-tropical areas, and are responsible for severe economic losses in livestock. The major losses, however, caused by ticks are due to their ability to transmit protozoan, rickettsial and viral diseases of livestock, which are of great economic importance world-wide.

Tick-borne protozoan diseases (e.g. Theileriosis and Babesiosis) and rickettsial diseases (e.g. Anaplasmosis) and cowdriosis and tick-associated dermatophilosis are major health and management problems of livestock in many developing countries.

The economically most important ixodid ticks of livestock in tropical regions belong to the genera of *Hyalomma*, *Boophilus*, *Rhipicephalus* and *Amblyomma* (Frans, 2000).

There are various ways to control ticks, but every method of tick control has certain shortcomings. Chemical control with acaricides was considered as one of the best methods, but it was shown recently that ticks have developed resistance against a range of acaricides (Martins et al., 1995).

However these chemicals are toxic and costly. Problems of acaricide resistance, chemical residues in food and the environment and the unsuitability of tick resistant cattle for all production systems make the current situation unsatisfactory, which is why there is debate on the development of an alternate and absolute control method, such as through vaccine.

Ticks have become an increasing problem to people and animals. Ticks are obligate blood-feeders that require an animal host to survive and reproduce.

They feed on a wide variety of mammals, birds, reptiles, and even amphibians. While most ticks feed on specific host animals and are not considered to be of medical or veterinary importance, several ticks have a wide host range and attack people, pets, or livestock.

Ticks can be a nuisance; their bites can cause irritation and, in the case of some ticks, paralysis. Severe infestations on animals can cause anemia, weight loss, and even death from the consumption of large quantities of blood. Ticks can also transmit many human and animal disease pathogens, which include viruses, bacteria, rickettsiae, and protozoa.

The association between ticks and disease was first demonstrated when Theobald Smith and Fred Kilbourne proved in 1893 that Texas cattle fever (cattle babesiosis) was caused by a protozoan transmitted by an infected tick.

In the late 1800s, Rocky Mountain spotted fever was the first human tick-borne disease identified in the United States, and for many years, was the major tick-associated disease in this country.

Although first recognized from the virulent cases in the Bitterroot Valley of Montana, it eventually became evident that most cases were distributed through the eastern United States.

Lyme disease was first recognized as a distinct clinical entity from a group of patients with arthritis in the area of Lyme, Connecticut, in 1975, although it became evident that this disease had an extensive history in Europe throughout the twentieth century. Today, Lyme disease is the leading arthropodˇ associated disease in the United States with nearly

24,000 human cases reported to the Centers for Disease Control and Prevention (CDC) in 2005.

This may represent only about 10% of physicianˇ diagnosed cases. Surveys have found that up to a quarter of residents in Lyme disease endemic areas have been diagnosed with the disease and that many residents perceive the disease as a serious or very serious problem. Without an effective intervention strategy, the steadily increasing trend in Lyme disease case reports is likely to continue.

In the northeastern United States, the emergence of Lyme disease can be linked to changing landscape patterns. A Swedish naturalist named Pehr Kalm recorded in his journal of his travels in the United States in 1748-1750 that ticks wereabundant and annoying.

Over a century later in 1872, entomologist Asa Fitch noted that ticks were nearly or quite extinct along the route that Pehr Kalm had traveled. During this time, the land had been cleared for agriculture and white-tailed deer in many areas were drastically reduced or virtually eliminated due to habitat loss and unregulated hunting.

With the reestablishment of forested habitat and animal hosts through the latter half of the twentieth century, ticks that may have survived on islands off the southern New England coast were able to increase and spread. The blacklegged tick, Ixodes scapularis, which is commonly known as the "deer" tick, and the principal vector for Lyme disease or Lyme borreliosis, was present on Naushon Island, Massachusetts, in the 1920s and 1930s. Some I. scapularis from Montauk Point, Long Island, New York, that were collected in the late 1940s and early 1950s were found infected with Lyme disease bacteria.

The risk of human infection increased through the 1960s and 1970s until the recognition of the disease from the cluster of cases in Lyme,

Connecticut, in 1975. Indeed, the disease was not new and cases had occurred in Europe through the 20th century under different names.

The rising incidence of Lyme disease is due to a number of factors including:

- Increased tick abundance
- Overabundant deer population
- Increased recognition of the disease
- Establishment of more residences in wooded areas
- Increased potential for contact with ticks.

With the steady increase in the incidence and geographic spread of Lyme disease, there is a need for homeowners, public health officials, and the pest control industry to learn how to manage or control the tick problem. The purpose of this handbook is to provide basic information on ticks and their biology, basic information on the diseases they carry, methods to reduce the risk of exposure to these parasites, and most importantly, information on how to reduce or manage tick populations, and therefore risk of disease, in the residential landscape.

Ticks are not insects but are arthropods more closely related to mites, spiders, scorpions, and harvestmen. There are about 80 species of ticks in the United States (~ 865 species worldwide). However, only about 12 or so in the U.S. are of major public health or veterinary importance with a few others that occasionally attack humans. The ticks discussed in this handbook belong to the family Ixodidae or hard ticks. The principal hard ticks recovered from humans in the mid-Atlantic and northeastern United States are the blacklegged (i.e., deer) tick, Ixodes scapularis, the American dog tick, Dermacentor variabilis, and the lone star tick, *Amblyomma americanum.*

Other tick species recorded as feeding on humans in the eastern U.S. include Ixodes cookei, Ixodes dentatus, and the brown dog tick, *Rhipicephalus sanguineus*.

The Argasidae or soft ticks form the other major group of ticks. Soft ticks are generally nest inhabitants that are associated with rodents, birds, or bats. Several species of soft ticks attack humans and can transmit disease organisms, mainly in western states, but are not the focus of this handbook. One species, Carios (Ornithodoros) kelleyi, a bat tick, has been recovered from states in the northeast, including Connecticut.

Scientific Names and a Few Terms

The scientific name of ticks, like other organisms, is given in two parts: genus (capitalized, often abbreviated by the first letter, e.g. I. scapularis) and species (not capitalized) sometimes followed by the name of the person who described the organism (given in parenthesis if the genus name is later changed).

The name Linneaus is abbreviated L. Common names like deer tick can vary regionally and some organisms may have no common name. The common names used in this guide follow those offi cially recognized by scientifi c societies. Several terms are used to defi ne the cycles of animal, tick and pathogen

Pathogen:

The microorganism (i.e., virus, bacteria, rickettsia, protozoa, fungus) that may cause disease.

• Parasite:

An animal that lives in or on a host for at least part of their life and benefits from the association at the expense of the host (from the Greek, literally para - beside and sitos - food).

• Vector:

An insect or other arthropod, like a tick, that carries and transmits a disease pathogen. Diseases associated with pathogens transmitted by a vector are called vectorˇ borne diseases.

• Host:

An animal infected by a pathogen or infested with a parasite. • Reservoir: An animal host that is capable of maintaining a pathogen and serving as a source of infection.

• Zoonoses:

A disease caused by a pathogen that is maintained in vertebrate animals that can be transmitted naturally to humans or domestic animals by a vector or through other means (e.g. saliva, feces). • Endemic disease: A disease that is established and present more or less continuously in a community.

Pesticides are commonly regarded as substances used to control organisms such as insects, fungi, weeds, and microbes that destroy plants, particularly those for food production.

They are also used for many other purposes, from public health campaigns against vector insects that cause devastating diseases such as malaria, typhus and dengue, to urban fumigation for hygienic purposes or home spraying to eliminate annoying bugs.

Today, a huge number of substances are employed as pesticides. The earliest pesticides included mineral compounds and extracts of natural products such as tobacco, chrysanthemum flower, or derris root.

During the second half of the nineteenth century, new products were introduced such as copper fungicides (the most famous being the Bordeaux mixture of copper sulphate and calcium hydroxide) and arsenic compounds (Paris Green and calcium and lead arsenate), which maintained their predominance until the first third of the twentieth century.8 In a popular book written at the end of the nineteenth century, a horticulturalist of the New York State Agricultural Experiment.

No one knows for certain the extent of the damage done to wildlife from the use of pesticides. This is because; no detailed study has been carried out to determine the real damage to fauna. However, many species have been affected, especially animals (Mason, et al., 1986) at the top of the food chain, and according to (Bramble, 1989) the natural balance of predators and prey has been disrupted, particularly in the insect world (Murray, A., 1985).

Birds, too, have been a casualty from pesticide poisoning(Lundholm, 1987) According to (Urfi, 1994) cranes and storks have been affected due to green revolution agricultural toxins. It is believed that agricultural toxins have decimated water insects and invertebrates in the agricultural lands that constitute up to 75% of Uttar Pradesh.

As a result, Sarus cranes, the world's largest flying bird, begun to disappear due to the disappearance of their specialized food. Storks, too, have been affected.

The number of Black Necked Storks have shown a visible decline and among the many factors responsible, have been the thinning of the shells of their eggs due to pesticides (Urfi, 1994).

There is a paucity of studies conducted to determine the welfare estimates of environmental effects of pesticides both in developed and developing countries despite the damage done to local flora and fauna being high.

Antle et al., 1994, 1994 a, &1998, have conducted an analysis of economic, environmental and health tradeoffs in Ecuador but the welfare estimates of environmental damages are not presented.

Pingali and Rosegrant (1994), too, discuss the environmental consequences of the green revolution in Asia but no welfare estimates of environmental damage are presented.

In Britain, Marchant et al. (1990), Department of the Environment (1996), have estimated that nine species of British farmland birds have experienced a serious decline between 25%-60% during the 1980's and that pesticide usage has been a significant factor.

Foster and Mourato (1997) have used this analysis to form the basis of their contingent ranking16 methodology to value the various environmental consequences of pesticide use in bread production. In this study three product attributes are considered, namely the price of a standard loaf of bread, causes of human illness as a result of field exposure to pesticides during cultivation and a number of farmland bird species in a state of serious long-term decline as a result of pesticide use in arable farming.

Tradeoffs between money, human morbidity and bird biodiversity are then examined. The willingness to pay valuation is expressed in terms of pence per loaf for a unit reduction of one case of ill health each year and one less bird species facing serious long-term decline.

The willingness to pay results show that to protect a bird species is typically six times higher (at around six pence per loaf) than the willingness to pay toenvironmental degradation.

Their contingent valuation survey was carried out among farmers in the USA. The results show that about 66% of the farmers were willing to pay to avoid environmental risks. The mean environmental cost estimates were $ 12.54 to avoid high risks, $8.76 to avoid moderate risks, $5.79 to avoid low risks (n= 1,114).

The cattle tick

The cattle tick, *Boophilus microplus,* is a significant ectoparasite of cattle and a vector for important diseases such as babesiosis and anaplasmosis.

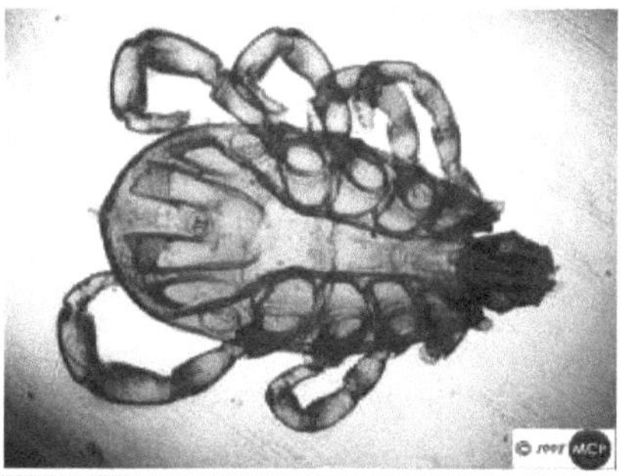

Boophilus microplus (male)

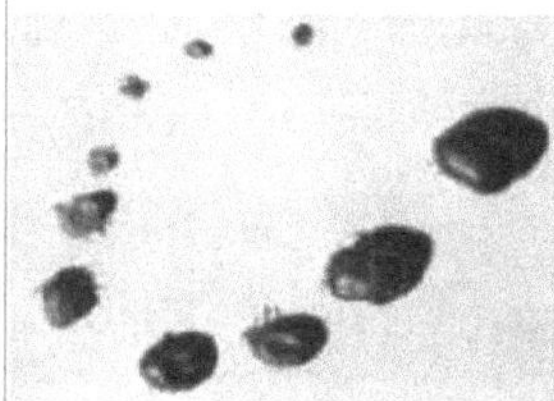

Life cycle of cattle tick.

Stages de développement de la tique du bétail.

Classification

SPC List D disease

Susceptible species

B. microplus is primarily a parasite of cattle. However, heavy infestations can also occur on horses, sheep, deer and water buffalo. Rarely, ticks have been reported on marsupials, goats, dogs, cats and pigs.

Distribution

The cattle tick is widely distributed in Central and South America, parts of the southern USA, Africa, Asia, and northern Australia. The distribution of the cattle tick is largely determined by climatic factors. *B. microplus* requires high humidity and ambient temperatures of at least 15-20o C for egg laying and hatching.

Clinical signs

Cattle tick infestation causes:

- Damage to hides
- Loss of production
- Anaemia and death
- Weakness leading to greater mortalities during droughts

Post-mortem findings

Animals may be in poor condition and anaemic. Infestations will be obvious by the presence of engorged ticks attached to the animal's skin.

Differential diagnosis

Several species of ticks may be found on cattle and it is important to differentiate these from *B. microplus*. Other ticks include:

- *Haemophysalis* spp
- *Ixodes holocyclus*

Specimens required for diagnosis

Ticks should be collected and forwarded to an entomologist for confirmation of the diagnosis. *B. microplus* has pale legs, short mouth parts with transversely ridged palps, small eyes and lacks an anal groove.

Transmission

The life cycle involves free-living stages. After feeding on cattle, engorged female ticks drop to the ground and lay eggs (up to 5000). After hatching, the larvae survive on pasture for several months.

The larvae then become quite active and climb up grass and transfer to animals as they brush past. The larvae attach and feed from the host. They moult to the nymphal stage and then undergo a further moult to the adult stage.

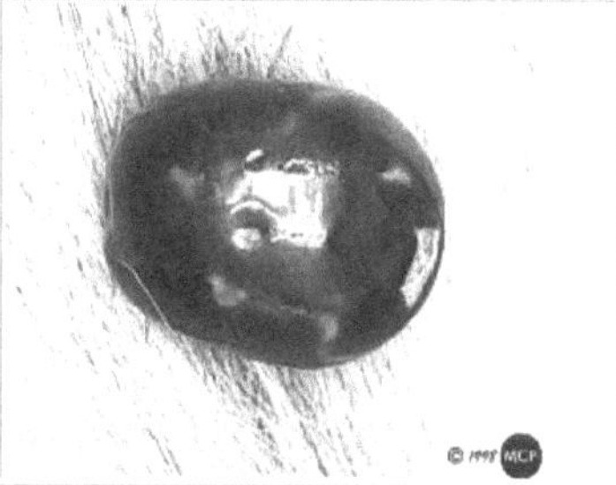	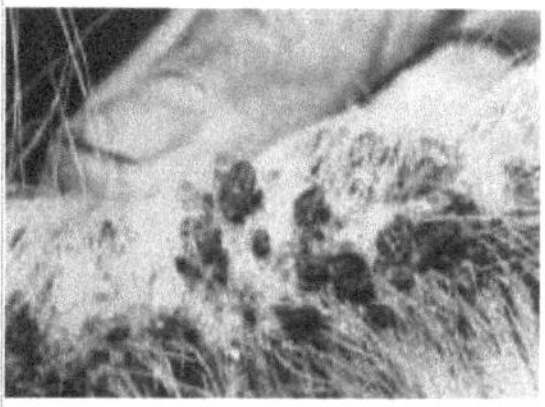
Engorged female, dorsal.	Heavy parasistim by cattle ticks.
Femelle engorgée, vue dorsale.	Impcrtant parasitisme par des tiques du bétail.

Photos Copyright FAO 1997

Risk of introduction

Cattle ticks are most likely to be introduced with the importation of infested cattle. Cattle tick was introduced to New Caledonia with cattle imported from Australia in this way.

Transport of ticks on dogs is considered a potential risk for introducing the tick to new areas, although egg production is much reduced in this species and the risk is considered low.

Control / vaccines

There are four methods available for controlling ticks:

- Treatment with acaricides
- Pasture spelling
- The use of resistant cattle
- Vaccination

Tick control by acaracide dipping has been widely used in endemic areas. Acaracides used for this purpose include various synthetic pyrethroids, amitraz, and some organophosphates. Dipping may have to be done as frequently as every 4-6 weeks in heavily infested areas. Many producers in tick endemic area have changed to *Bos indicus* type cattle because of their greater resistance to tick infection.

An anti-tick vaccine is also commercially available in Australia. The vaccine antigen, based on a tick gut protein and produced by recombinant technology, stimulates production of specific antibodies in cattle which damage the gut of engorging ticks, resulting in a fertility reduction of up to 70% in adult ticks, reducing tick population build-up. This vaccine is of limited use, but can be used as part of an integrated program for the control of ticks

Cattle ticks (*Rhipicephalus microplus*) are the most serious external parasite of cattle in northern Australia. They transmit tick fever and if uncontrolled, can cause serious losses to the cattle industry.

HOSTS

Engorged female Adult female although cattle ticks favour cattle, infestations occur on buffaloes, deer, camels, horses and sheep. Cattle ticks may occasionally be seen on donkeys, goats, dogs and pigs. When cattle are heavily infested, ticks can be found anywhere on the body. On lightly infested animals, the main places to look for ticks are the escutcheon, tail butt, belly, shoulder, dewlap and ear.

EFFECTS

Infested cattle lose condition due to 'tick worry' and loss of blood. Heavy infestations can kill calves and even adult cattle. Animals in poor condition are especially vulnerable. Previously unexposed cattle become heavily infested until they build up a degree of resistance.

Bos indicus (tropical breeds of cattle) and their crosses, develop a greater degree of resistance than do Bos taurus (British and European breeds of cattle).

Cattle ticks transmit the organisms that cause tick fever, which is a serious blood parasite disease of cattle. The disease can be lethal to susceptible animals. Others may suffer severe loss of condition. Hides of infested cattle are damaged by tick bites, reducing their value. In severe cases the hides may be unsaleable.

Horses also suffer from ‘tick worry’ and loss of blood from cattle tick infestations. They rub and bite affected areas, causing severe skin lesions. After a period, however, horses develop strong resistance to cattle ticks. Cattle ticks have little effect on other hosts.

SEASONAL DISTRIBUTION

In the Northern Territory (NT), cattle ticks can be seen at any time of the year, but mainly occur during the wet season and early dry season.

IDENTIFYING CATTLE TICKS

All three parasitic stages are generally present on infested cattle, but the easiest to identify is the adult stage. Cattle ticks are the only ticks with all legs that are a pale cream in colour.

SPECIMENS

Larvae, nymphs or unfed adults should be put in a bottle with three parts methylated spirit and one part water. Engorged adult ticks should be put live on blotting paper, covered with moist cotton wool and put into a screw-top bottle with small holes for ventilation. Live adult females are required for testing for resistance to insecticides.

It is most important to provide the name and address of the property and the date the specimens were collected. As labels may become detached, lost, or illegible, identification notes should be written on a piece of paper in pencil, which is not affected by methylated spirit, and put in the specimen bottle or jar. Packages containing methylated spirit or live ticks must not be sent by post, air or bus.

RESISTANT TICKS

Ticks can be killed by dipping or spraying cattle with an appropriate chemical (acaricide). Ticks can, however, develop resistance to acaricides. Larvae produced by engorged adult females are tested for acaricide resistance at a laboratory in Brisbane. Contact your local Livestock Biosecurity Officer if you suspect acaricide resistance.

CONTROL

Cattle ticks can be controlled by using resistant cattle, strategic treatment with chemicals, pasture spelling or a combination of these methods. In the NT, cattle ticks are usually controlled by using resistant cattle; treatment is usually limited to cattle awaiting export or moving to or through tick-free areas.

LIFE CYCLE

There are four stages in the life cycle of cattle ticks. Cattle ticks are one host ticks, that is, the larva, nymph and adult remain on the same animal. The parasitic phase of the life cycle lasts about three weeks.

The life cycle consists of two parts, the parasitic part during which ticks feed on cattle, and the non-parasitic part during which they spend on the ground. © Northern Territory Government Page 2 of 4 Parasitic part of the life cycle When 'seed' ticks (larvae) infest a host they usually bite immediately and begin feeding.

However, during the first two days following infestation, feeding is intermittent and the larvae frequently detach to move about on the host. After five to six days, they ingest a large meal of tissue fluids and blood, and moult to become eight-legged nymphs. Nymphs also feed on the host's blood and moult to young adults after six to eight days.

Males usually moult first and can be found lying underneath engorged nymphs and female ticks. Males are much smaller and more active than females. The parasitic life of ticks is completed eight to 12 days after the nymphal moult.

The full life cycle is completed in 19 to 26 days. Fully engorged male ticks may either remain on the host or detach with the female. Males have been known to survive for 70 days, either on the host, or on vegetation, relying on dew or plant juices for their fluid needs.

Non-parasitic part of the life cycle This begins when the fully engorged female tick, in the stage during which it is most easily seen on infested cattle, falls to the ground and finds a suitable place to lay eggs.

The pre-egg laying period depends on environmental temperature and relative humidity, and can be as short as one to two days or as long as 40 days. The duration of egg-laying is also temperature-controlled and can range from two to 44 days. Each female tick may lay up to 3500 eggs.

During the wet season when both temperature and humidity are optimal, eggs hatch in approximately 18 to 21 days. © Northern Territory Government Page 3 of 4 The six-legged larvae which hatch from the eggs are known as seed ticks. They are extremely active in response to moving objects.

The close proximity of an animal is sufficient to activate them to climb to the tips of blades of grass, where they can attach more easily to a passing host. During the evening, seed ticks seek protection in the vegetation. The longevity of seed ticks is influenced by temperature and humidity.

They are extremely vulnerable to very low ambient temperatures and low humidity. In northern Australia the maximum longevity is two to four months depending on the season. The non-parasitic part of the life cycle ends when seed ticks find suitable hosts. These may not necessarily be cattle. Cattle ticks have been known to infest horses, sheep, dogs, buffalo, deer, pigs and hares, although cattle are the preferred host.

Tick ecology

Chaka et al.(2001) studied determination of the physiological age of *Rhipicephalus appendiculatus*. The age structure of a population of vectors of disease pathogens is a most useful characteristic for epidemiological studies.

It has long been developed for insect vectors, where the success of an eradication programme can be plotted by the declining survival. Age grading of ticks requires theoretical adaptation because of the fundamentally different relationship between feeding and transmission opportunities of insect and ticks.

Estrada-Peña (2001) reported that seasonal dynamics exert a major influence on the dynamics of transmission of tick-born pathogen.

Tick Biology and Behavior

Ticks, like many mite species, are obligate blood-feeders, requiring a host animal for food and development. Ticks have four stages in their life cycle: egg, the 6-legged larva (seed ticks), and 8-legged nymph and adult (male or female).

Larvae and nymphs change to the next stage after digesting a blood meal by molting or shedding the cuticle. Most of the ticks mentioned in this handbook have a 3-host life cycle, whereas each of the three active stages feed on a different individual host animal, taking a single blood meal. Larvae feed to repletion on one animal, drop to the ground and molt to a nymph.

The nymphs must find and attach to another animal, engorge, drop to ground and molt to an adult. The adult tick feeds on a third animal. A replete or engorged (blood filled) female tick will produce a single large batch of eggs and then die. Depending upon the species of tick, egg mass deposited can range roughly from 1,000 to 18,000 eggs.

3-host tick life cycle 8 Stafford The Connecticut Agricultural Experimentation Station Bulletin No. 1010 5 The larvae and nymphs generally feed on small to medium-sized hosts, while adult ticks feed on larger animals. Some ticks may have one-host (all stages staying and feeding on only one animal host before the female drops off) or other multi-host lifecycles. Depending upon the tick, the life cycle may be completed in 1, 2 or even 3 years, while a one-host tick may have more than one generation per year. Feeding for only a few days, the majority of the life of a tick is spent off the host in the environment either seeking a host, molting or simply passing through an inhospitable season (e.g., hot summers or cold winters).

Soft ticks have a multi-host life cycle with multiple nymphal stages; each stage feeds briefly, and adults take multiple small blood meals, laying small egg batches after each feeding. As nest and cave dwellers, often with transient hosts, some argasid ticks may survive many years without a host.

However, most hard ticks do not successfully fi nd a host and perish within months or a year or two at best. Larval ticks will be clustered on the egg mass after hatching and when ready to feed, ascend blades of grass or similar vegetation to await a host.

Ticks assume a questing position by clinging to the leaf litter or vegetation with the third and fourth pair of legs, and hold the first pair outstretched. Due to differences in susceptibility to desiccation and host preference, immature ticks generally remain in the low vegetation, while adult ticks may seek a host at a higher level in the vegetation.

Ticks detect their hosts through several host odors (including carbon dioxide, ammonia, lactic acid, and other specific body odors), body heat, moisture, vibrations, and for some, visual cues like a shadow.

When approached by a potential host, a tick becomes excited - waving the front legs in order to grab the passing host. Ticks cannot fl y or jump; they must make direct contact with a host.

Once on a host a tick may attach quickly or wander over the host for some time. Some ticks attach only or principally on certain areas like the ear or thin-skinned areas, while other species may attach almost anywhere on the host. The ticks feed slowly, remaining on the host for several days, until engorged with blood (see following section on tick feeding).

Male ticks feed intermittently, take small blood meals, and may remain on a host for weeks. For most ticks mating occurs on the host, as the male tick also requires a blood meal. However, male Ixodes ticks do not need to feed prior to mating and mating may occur on or off the host.

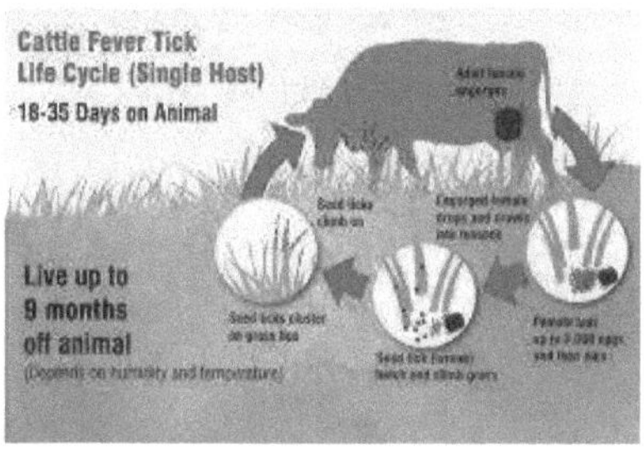

Cattle fever ticks

Tick Morphology

The body of a tick consists of a "false head" (the capitulum) and a thorax and abdomen fused into a single oval, flattened body. A larval tick has six legs, while nymphs and adults have eight legs present. The basal segment of the leg, the coxa, may have spurs that help in identifi cation.

An adult tick will have a genital aperture on the ventral surface, located roughly between the second pair of legs. The respiratory system is evident by spiracular plates located ventrolaterally behind the fourth pair of legs in the nymphs and adults.

These plates may be oval, rounded, or comma-shaped. Hard ticks get their name from a tough dorsal shield or plate called the scutum present on all mobile stages of the tick. The scutum on the larva, nymph, and female tick covers the dorsal anterior third to half of the body. By contrast, the scutum on a male tick covers almost the entire dorsal surface and expansion during feeding is very limited.

The scutum differs in shape and others characteristics (i.e., presence or absence of simple eyes) between tick genera. In some ticks, ornate or patterned markings may be present that can aid in identification. A distinct semicircular anal groove curves around the front of the anal opening in Ixodes ticks.

In all other ticks, the anal groove is behind the anus or absent. Many ticks, but not Ixodes, have rectangular areas separated by grooves on the posterior margin of the tick body called festoons. Festoons, if present, may not be visible on fully engorged females. Argasid ticks are leathery, wrinkled and grayish in appearance. The capitulum of soft ticks is located on the underside of the body and cannot be seen from above.

The capitulum in hard ticks is visible dorsally in all stages. The capitulum holds the mouthparts consisting of a base (basis capituli), two palps, paired chelicerae, and the median ventral hypostome, which is covered with denticles or recurved teeth.

The shape of the basis capituli, length of the palps, number of denticles, and other characteristics of the mouthparts are used to help identify tick genera and species. While the adults of some common ticks can be easily identified with a little training because of distinctive markings or color, the identification of most ticks and the immature stages requires the services of a trained entomologist and the use of keys developed by tick taxonomists.

These keys are designed to specifi cally identify adults, nymphs or larvae. Above right: Mouthparts of I. scapularis nymphs showing hypostome with rows of denticles (center) and two pair chelicerae (palps are partially visible).

How a Tick Feeds

The term tick bite may be misleading as ticks do not bite and depart or feed rapidly like a mosquito. Ticks attach and feed gradually over a period of several to many days. Once a tick has found a suitable place to feed, it grasps the skin, tilts the body at a 45-60° angle, and begins to cut into the skin with the paired chelicerae.

The palps lay outwards on the skin surface. After the chelicerae and hypostome penetrate the skin, they become encased in "cement" secreted by the tick. The cement serves to hold the mouthparts in place while the tick feeds.

Mouthparts on larval and nymphal ticks are small with less penetration and produce a smaller host reaction. Adult Ixodes and Amblyomma ticks have long mouthparts that can reach the subdermal layer of skin, produce a larger reaction, and make the tick harder to remove. Insertion of the mouthparts often takes around 10-30 minutes, but can take longer (1-2 hours).

The reaction to a feeding tick may make the tick appear imbedded, but only the slender mouthparts actually penetrate the skin.

Physical and enzymatic rupture of tissue creates a lesion or cavity under the skin from which blood is imbibed. A variety of pharmacologically active compounds that aid the feeding process and possibly increase pathogen transmission are introduced in the tick's saliva (e.g., blood platelet aggregation inhibitors, anticoagulants, anti-infl ammatory and immunosuppressive agents, enzymes, and vasodilators to increase blood flow).

Feeding is not continuous and most of the blood meal is taken up during the last 12-24 hours of feeding. The body weight of a feeding female tick can increase 80-120 times. Male ticks are intermittent feeders, take smaller amounts of blood, and do not change appreciably in size (male I. scapularis do not need to feed and are rarely found attached).

Ticks may attach and feed anywhere on the body, but there are differences depending upon exposure and species of tick. The distribution of the blacklegged tick is relatively uniform. However, over a third of I. scapularis were from the legs and arms and another third were from the back up through the shoulders, neck and head. By contrast, most American dog ticks are removed from the head and neck region.

The Blacklegged Tick or "Deer" Tick, Ixodes scapularis Say

Blacklegged tick is the correct common name for the tick popularly known as the "deer" tick (the terms are not used together, it is not called the blacklegged deer tick).

Ixodes (pronounced x-zod-ease) scapularis transmits the causal agents of three diseases; Lyme disease, human babesiosis, and human granulocytic anaplasmosis (HGA). The northern range of the tick includes southern portions of Canada and coastal Maine through the mid-Atlantic states into Maryland, Delaware and northern parts of Virginia and in several north central states, particularly Wisconsin and Minnesota, extending down through Illinois and into Indiana.

This tick is also found throughout the southeastern United States west to southcentral Texas, Oklahoma, southern Missouri, and eastern Kansas. However, few I. scapularis in the southeast have been found infected with the bacterium that causes Lyme disease, the spirochete Borrelia burgdorferi.

Therefore, the risk for Lyme disease from this tick in the southeastern United States is considered relatively low. Unfed female I. scapularis have a reddish body and a dark brown dorsal scutum (plate) located behind the mouthparts.

Length of the female tick from the tip of the palpi to the end of the body is about 3 to 3.7 mm (about 1/10 of an inch). Male I. scapularis are smaller (2 – 2.7 mm) than the female and are completely dark brown. Nymphs are 1.3 to 1.7 mm in length, while larvae are only 0.7 to 0.8 mm. Female blacklegged ticks become fairly large when engorged with blood and, consequently, are sometimes confused with engorged female American dog ticks.

The Blacklegged Tick or "Deer" Tick, Ixodes scapularis Say Blacklegged ticks feed on a wide variety of mammals and birds, requiring 3-7 days to ingest the blood, depending on the stage of the tick. Larvae and nymphs of I. scapularis typically become infected with B. burgdorferi when they feed on a reservoir competent host. The white-footed mouse is the principal reservoir (source of infection) for *B. burgdorferi*, the protozoan agent of human babesisois, Babesia microti, and can serve as a reservoir for the agent of human granulocytic ehrlichiosis. Birds are also a major host for immature I. scapularis and have been implicated in the long-distance dispersal of ticks and *B. burgdorferi*.

White-tailed deer, Odocoileus virginianus (Zimmerman), are the principal host for the adult stage of the tick, which feeds on a variety of medium- to large-sized mammalian hosts. An engorged female tick may typically lay around 2,000-3,000 eggs.

The Lyme disease spirochete in northern states is maintained, in part, by the two-year life cycle of the tick. Eggs are laid by the female in

May. Larvae hatch from those eggs in mid- to late July with August being the peak month for larval tick activity.

After feeding, the larvae drop from the host and molt to nymphs, which will appear the following year in late spring. May, June and July are peak months for nymphal tick activity in the northeast. Therefore, the nymphs precede larvae seasonally and can infect a new generation of animal hosts.

Larvae active later in the summer then become infected when feeding on reservoir host animals. The nymphal ticks will molt to adults after feeding and appear in the fall of the same year. Adult I. scapularis do not hibernate and may be active on warm winter days and the following spring. Adults of I. scapularis are more heavily infected with B. burgdorferi than the nymphs because the tick has had two opportunities to become infected, once as a larva and once as a nymph.

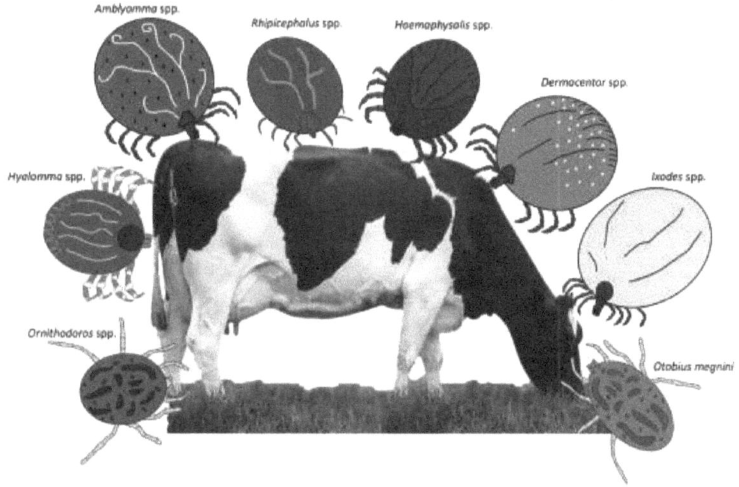

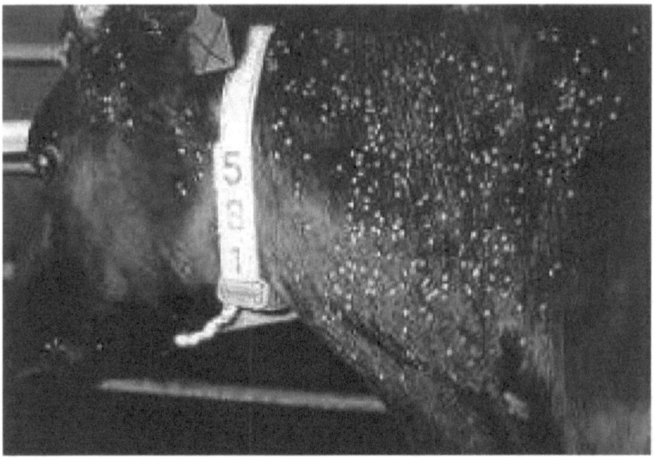

The ileria or tick disease

Tick Control

The main reasons for tick control are to protect hosts from irritation and production losses, formation of lesions that can become secondarily infested, damage to hides and udders, toxicosis, paralysis, and of greatest importance, infection with a wide variety of disease agents. Control also prevents the spread of tick species and the diseases they transmit to unaffected areas, regions, or continents.

Cultural and Biologic Control

These measures can be directed against both the free-living and parasitic stages of ticks. The free-living stages of most tick species, both ixodid and argasid, have specific requirements in terms of microclimate and are restricted to particular microhabitats within the ecosystems inhabited by their hosts.

Destruction of these microhabitats reduces the abundance of ticks. Alteration of the environment by removal of certain types of vegetation has been used in the control of *Amblyomma americanum* in recreational areas in southeastern USA and in the control of *Ixodes rubicundus* in South Africa.

Control of argasid ticks such as *Argas persicus* and *A walkerae* in poultry can be achieved by eliminating cracks in walls and perches, which provide shelter to the free-living stages.

The abundance of tick species can also be reduced by removal of alternative hosts or hosts of a particular stage of the life cycle. This approach has occasionally been advocated for control of three-host ixodid ticks such as *Rhipicephalus appendiculatus*, *Amblyomma hebraeum*, and *Ixodes rubicundus* in Africa, and *Hyalomma* spp in southeastern Europe and Asia.

Rotation of pastures or pasture spelling has been used in control of the one-host ixodid tick *Rhipicephalus (Boophilus) microplus* in Australia. The method could also be applied to other one-host ticks, in which the duration of the spelling period is determined by the relatively short life span of the free-living larvae. However, it has minimal application to multihost ixodid ticks or argasid ticks because of the long survival periods of the unfed nymphs and adults.

Predators, including birds, rodents, shrews, ants, and spiders, play a role in some areas in reducing the numbers of free-living ticks. In the New World, fire ants (*Pheidole megacephala*) are noteworthy tick predators. Engorged ticks may also become parasitized by the larvae of some wasps (Hymenoptera), but these have not significantly reduced tick populations.

Zebu (*Bos indicus*) and Sanga (a *B taurus*, *B indicus* crossbreed) cattle, the indigenous breeds of Asia and Africa, usually become very resistant to ixodid ticks after initial exposure. In contrast, European (*B taurus*) breeds usually remain fairly susceptible.

The tick resistance of Zebu breeds and their crosses is being increasingly exploited as a means of control of the parasitic stages. The introduction of Zebu cattle to Australia has revolutionized the control of *R microplus* on that continent.

Use of resistant cattle as a means of tick control is also becoming important in Africa and the Americas. In Africa, infestations of ixodid ticks on livestock and wild ungulates may also be reduced by oxpeckers (*Buphagus* spp), which are birds that feed on attached ticks.

Tick-Host Physical Interface

The cattle tick *R. microplus* co-evolved with Asian bovines (zebu breeds) and due to the global migration of *B. t. taurus* European breeds for dairy production during the eighteenth–nineteenth centuries, this tick spread across tropical and sub-tropical regions of the world (Frisch, 1999; Estrada-Peña et al., 2006; Barré and Uilenberg, 2010).

Currently *R. microplus* is considered to be a species complex, in which there are recognized geographic differences between the 5 clades including 3 clades of *R. microplus* (A, B, and C), as well as *R. australis* and *R. annulatus* (Burger et al., 2014; Low et al., 2015).

Each taxa transmits both anaplasmosis and babesiosis and each have a parasitic life cycle on cattle for ~21 days. They will be described collectively as *R. microplus* or simply as cattle ticks in this review. Cattle ticks are attracted to their hosts through stimuli such as carbon dioxide, temperature, vibrations, visual stimuli, and odor (Osterkamp et al., 1999).

The susceptible European (*B. t. taurus*) breeds which were introduced into regions in which *R. microplus* is endemic failed to resist tick infestation to the same extent as tropical *B. t. indicus* breeds, which have developed an effective anti-tick immune response (Frisch, 1999).

The immune response varies among newly introduced European cattle (Taurine breeds, susceptible hosts) whereas Asian bovines (zebuine breeds or resistant hosts) co-evolved with ticks (Utech et al., 1978).

Physical barriers that affect tick resistance include density of the fur coat, skin thickness, skin pigmentation (light or dark), skin vibration and/or self-cleaning ability, tongue papillae, and odor (de Castro et al., 1985; Spickett et al., 1989; Veríssimo et al., 2002, 2015; Martinez et al., 2006; Gasparin et al., 2007).

In addition to physical differences between resistant and susceptible hosts, their behavior also affects the *R. microplus* parasitic load. Self-grooming is widely used by cattle as an important defense mechanism against ticks (Riek, 1956; Snowball, 1956; Bennett, 1969) and the level of resistance may possibly be associated with tongue morphology.

For example the papillae from tick-resistant breeds have smaller spacing, which is more effective in removing *R. microplus* larvae from the skin (Veríssimo et al., 2015).

However, there is also conjecture that resistant breeds simply groom more often (Kemp et al., 1976). It has been suggested that innate characteristics such as thinner coats and lower fur density have direct impacts in decreasing tick preferential attachment and infestation (Spickett et al., 1989; Veríssimo et al., 2002; Gasparin et al., 2007; Marufu et al., 2011).

However, other studies have shown that skin features have no influence on tick infestation (Wagland, 1978; Doube and Wharton, 1980). Evidence for resistance of cattle to ticks due to physical parameters is scarce and further studies to examine the mechanisms that govern these physical phenomena are still needed.

Immunological Determinants Associated with Host Resistance: Host Counter Attack

It is well-established that cattle have three subclasses of IgG (IgG1, IgG2, and IgG3), and during blood meals ticks ingest a substantial amount of IgG (Knight et al., 1988; Symons et al., 1989; Kacskovics and Butler, 1996; Rabbani et al., 1997; Gudderra et al., 2002; Saini et al., 2007).

Host IgGs can be found in the tick hemolymph and are potentially biologically active against specific tick proteins (Ben-Yakir et al., 1987). Furthermore, specific host antibodies neutralize the tick salivary pharmacopeia and can damage the tick by binding to tick internal organs such as salivary glands, midgut, or ovaries (Ackerman et al., 1981; Willadsen and Kemp, 1988; Tellam et al., 1992).

In other tick-host systems (*Dermacentor andersoni* and guinea pigs), antibodies have been shown to mediate inflammatory reactions by triggering effector-cell recruitment and cellular immune response as a consequence of both Fc receptor activation of leukocytes and complement activation that are harmful to the tick, also an immune mechanism in human auto-immune disease syndromes (Wikel and Whelen, 1986; Hogarth, 2002).

It was documented previously that the passive transfer of plasma from genetically immune resistant animals to naïve hosts, increases resistance to tick challenge and this response was believed to be mediated by antibodies (Roberts and Kerr, 1976; Shapiro et al., 1986).

The pattern of antibody responses to immunogens from tick salivary glands and guts have been reviewed by different research groups

(Willadsen, 1980; Wikel, 1982; Kaufman, 1989; Kashino et al., 2005; Cruz et al., 2008; Piper et al., 2009, 2010; Garcia et al., 2017).

Some studies have shown that during laboratory animal infestations, such as guinea pigs, rabbits and mice, reactive antibody titers to tick salivary antigens increased (Allen and Humphreys, 1979; Allen, 1989).

The densities of *Amblyomma hebraeum, Rhipicephalus appendiculatus*, and *Rhipicephalus evertsi evertsi* ticks was higher on the susceptible breed (*B. t. taurus* Hereford) as compared to resistant cattle (*B. t. indicus* Brahman) with a positive correlation between the level of tick infestation and the level of IgG in susceptible hosts (Rechav, 1987).

Piper and colleagues confirmed this correlation noting that susceptible cattle (Holstein-Friesian) have higher levels of tick specific IgGs compared to Brahmans suggesting that these antibodies do not confer immunity to ticks (Piper et al., 2008, 2009, 2010).

As with other immune parameters in high and low resistance animals, the interpretation of data can be problematic as a susceptible animal will have more ticks feeding at any time, which would in turn be expected to result in a higher antigenic challenge.

However, the negative relationship between IgG levels and host resistance was later confirmed and shown to be independent of the number of feeding ticks, using Santa Gertrudis cattle [a stable composite breed of *B. t. taurus* (5/8) and *B. t. indicus* (3/8)], in which there is wide variation in host resistance to ticks (Piper et al., 2017).

Susceptible animals had significantly higher tick-specific IgG1 antibody titres (to several tick antigens including adult female salivary glands and guts, and whole larvae) compared to tick resistant cattle (Piper et al., 2017). In contrast, Kashino et al reported that tick saliva-specific IgG1 and IgG2 antibodies decreased in susceptible (Holstein) compared to resistant (Nelore) cattle where the IgG levels remained the same, however, only IgG levels to tick salivary antigens were examined (Kashino et al., 2005). Previous studies have surmised that there are genetic differences in the bovine host's ability to elicit antibody responses to antigens in *R. microplus* and *D. andersoni* tick saliva (Whelen et al., 1986; Opdebeeck and Daly, 1990). Despite the fact that differences in the IgG levels against tick antigens between heavy or light infestations have been reported, there is individual variation in the same bovine breed with respect to humoral immune responses to tick antigenic molecules (Cruz et al., 2008). In addition, despite most studies reporting increased total IgG production against wide ranging tick antigens in susceptible breeds compared to resistant, IgG responses to salivary proteins were significantly higher in tick naïve resistant hosts (Nelore) at the first larval challenge (Garcia et al., 2017).

Variation in IgG2 allotypes has been associated with variation in immune responses to pathogens. When two allotypes IgG2a and IgG2b were found to differ in sequence at the CH1–CH3 regions it was reported that IgG2b was more able to initiate the bovine complement cascade while animals with the IgG2a allotype were more susceptible to extracellular pyogenic pathogens (Heyermann and Butler, 1987; Bastida-Corcuera et al., 1999). Other studies have shown that the distribution and presence of IgG2 allotypes differed significantly between taurine and indicine breeds (Butler et al., 1994; Carvalho et al., 2011). Blakeslee et al. (1971) described that ~80% of susceptible bovines (Holstein) have the IgG2a allotype and that the IgGγ2b was rare in these animals (Blakeslee et al., 1971). Recently, it was shown that the IgGγ2a allotype was significantly more frequent in taurine hosts (tick susceptible) and IgGγ2b was significantly frequent in indicine cattle (tick resistant) (Carvalho et al., 2011). Male tick saliva contains IgG-binding proteins (IGBPs) secreted into the host which assists the female tick to evade the host immune response (Wang and Nuttall, 1999; Santos et al., 2004; Gong et al., 2014). Carvalho et al. (2011) suggested that certain IgG2 allotypes may hinder the function of these tick IGBPs.

Aside from IGBPs, other tick specific proteins have been examined in terms of their immune recognition by tick resistant and susceptible cattle. A *R. microplus* recombinant serine protease inhibitor (Serpin- rRMS-3) was recognized by resistant bovines and not susceptible, suggesting that RMS-3 could be a protective antigen (Rodriguez-Valle et al., 2012).

Another study by the same group demonstrated that host responses to six *R. microplus* lipocalins (LRMs which include tick histamine binding proteins) were higher in resistant cattle (Rodriguez-Valle et al., 2013).

Both RMS-3 and the LRM proteins were identified based on the *in silico* identification of B cell binding epitopes. In addition, predicted T cell epitopes from 3 LRMs stimulated the generation of a significantly higher number of interferon gamma (IFN-γ) secreting cells (consistent with a Th1 response) in tick-susceptible Holstein–Friesians compared with tick-resistant Brahman cattle. In contrast, expression of the Th2-associated cytokine interleukin-4 (IL4) was lower in Holstein–Friesian (susceptible) cattle when compared with Brahman (resistant) cattle (Rodriguez-Valle et al., 2013).

IL4 is known to decrease the production of Th1 cells and IFN-γ, and is thus a key regulator of both the humoral and adaptive immune responses.

The immunological parameters of tick resistance have been shown to differ between tick susceptible and tick resistant breeds as well as within the same breeds. The studies reported differ in the parameters of trials and tick infestations, for example, the use of tick naïve cattle artificially infested or the use of cattle naturally exposed to ticks (Kashino et al., 2005; Piper et al., 2008, 2009). The study undertaken by Kashino et al. (2005) used susceptible cattle that had been treated with acaricides when high tick numbers were observed and the cattle had been vaccinated with GAVAC (Bm86 based tick vaccine), introducing additional variables to the study. Further studies examining specific tick proteins to compare divergent host immune responses are still warranted.

Molecular Genetic Variants Associated with Host Resistance

Numerous studies have attempted to identify genetic markers for host resistance to tick infestation and they are summarized and discussed by Porto Neto et al. (2011b) and Mapholi et al. (2014).

Approaches have included immunological methods (Stear et al., 1984, 1989, 1990); protein-based analyses (Ashton et al., 1968; Carvalho et al., 2008); candidate gene sequence or genotype (Acosta-Rodriguez et al., 2005; Martinez et al., 2006; Untalan et al., 2007); genomic detection of quantitative trait loci (QTL) using SNPs or microsatellites, with or without fine mapping (Barendse, 2007; Gasparin et al., 2007; Regitano et al., 2008; Prayaga et al., 2009; Machado et al., 2010; Porto Neto et al., 2010a, 2011a; Turner et al., 2010; Cardoso et al., 2015; Mapholi et al., 2016; Sollero et al., 2017).

There is one example of a meta-analysis of genomic association with transcriptome in tick infestation (Porto Neto et al., 2010b). Although this appears to represent a large body of science, it has generated relatively little data which can be used for improved genetic selection. It can be concluded from the studies on the major histocompatibility complex (MHC, also referred to as the bovine lymphocyte antigen (BoLA) system) that the MHC makes a contribution to variation in resistance however there is no single, consistent genotype of any gene in the MHC that is associated with high or low resistance to ticks across breeds and production systems.

A number of QTL markers have been identified using microsatellites and SNPs, however these have mostly been inconsistent and the loci have had relatively weak effects. The research of Barendse (2007) and Turner et al. (2010) found several significant loci but most of them had effects in the order of 1% of the phenotypic variation in tick infestation. The lack of consistent and strong findings is not surprising. Counting ticks is difficult and time consuming thus studies resort to scoring systems, which are less precise than counts, and this can have an effect on heritability.

Alternatively, the numbers used tend to be relatively small and studies are underpowered. The most robust report is that by Turner et al. (2010), who reported on a study in which ticks were counted and heritability was a respectable 37%, and which used 1,960 cattle. In contrast, Prayaga et al. (2009) used a scoring system, 900 animals and estimated heritability of tick score to be 9%.

Furthermore, a study examining the genomic prediction for tick resistance in Braford (Brahman x Hereford/tick resistant x tick susceptible breed, respectively) and Hereford cattle in Brazil showed that genomic selection for tick resistant Braford cattle may be achievable (Cardoso et al., 2015).

A recent trait tag-SNP approach by the same group reported 914 SNPs explaining more than 20% of the estimated genetic variance for tick resistance (Sollero et al., 2017).

Despite the challenges of the genomic approach to identifying either mechanisms or markers for host resistance to ticks in cattle, they have enabled the identification of allelic variation in genes that are very likely to influence the trait. The *ELTD1* gene (EGF, latrophilin, and seven transmembrane domain containing 1) was identified from GWAS in dairy and beef cattle (Prayaga et al., 2009; Turner et al., 2010).

Its association with the host resistance phenotype was confirmed but its effect was limited to <1% of the total phenotypic variation in the trait (Porto Neto et al., 2011a).

Similarly, haplotypes that included the *ITGA11* gene (integrin alpha 11) were significantly associated with tick burden and explained about 1.5% of the variation in the trait. Finally, the potential functional role of allelic variation in a gene identified by the same GWAS studies (Prayaga et al., 2009; Turner et al., 2010) *RIPK2* (serine-threonine kinase 2) was further examined using knock out mice (Porto Neto et al., 2012).

This gene is known to play an essential role in the modulation of innate and adaptive immune responses and it was found that it influenced the recognition of tick salivary antigens by mice.

Limited association of tick burden or phenotype to the genotype is currently available and large bovine genomic meta-analyses may contribute to the identification of within breed markers for tick resistance in the future.

Variation in Gene Expression among Resistant and Susceptible Hosts and Relationship with Immune Responses

Bioactive molecules secreted by *R. microplus* ticks into the skin of the host during attachment and blood feeding stimulate host effective responses. The variation in the mechanisms by which each host breed responds to each of these bioactive molecules likely results in different levels of resistance.

It is well-established that the resistance to tick infestation is due to a complex set of responses, however the specific mechanisms and their relative importance continues to be the subject of debate.
Table 1 summarizes selected up-regulated genes including those that are potentially associated with immune responsiveness, blood coagulation, calcium regulation, and/or wound healing from several studies undertaken to date.

The parameters of all of the studies differ from each other including: the number of biological replicates, the number of larvae used in infestations, the breeds and subspecies used, their prior exposure, the methodology and platform used to measure host responses (immunohistochemistry, microarray platforms, qPCR), the timing of sample collection, and the samples analyzed (skin or blood). Without undertaking a formal meta-analysis of the original data, we have attempted to summarize differences and similarities in relation to susceptible vs. resistant animals among reports.

Studies on PBL suggest that resistant hosts are more likely to develop a stable T-cell-mediated response against *R. microplus*, while susceptible cattle demonstrated cellular and gene expression profiles consistent with innate and inflammatory responses to tick infestation (Kashino et al., 2005; Piper et al., 2009).

The up-regulation of genes in tick susceptible cattle involved in inflammatory and other important immunological responses mediate a greater natural potential to develop higher pro-inflammatory responses in comparison to tick resistant animals.

Gene expression studies on skin taken from larval attachment sites have demonstrated that cytokines, chemokines, and complement factors were differentially expressed between naïve-skin and infested skin in susceptible Holstein–Friesian cattle. It was also found that immunoglobulin transcripts were differentially expressed in infested skin from Holstein-Friesian compared to resistant Brahman cattle. Therefore, the chronic pathology established in *B. t. taurus* cattle might facilitate the tick feeding process (Piper et al., 2010).

In addition, extracellular matrix genes such as: keratocan, osteoglycin, collagen, and lumican were up-regulated in infested-skin from *B. t. indicus* resistant Brahman cattle. In a study involving coagulation in skin from resistant and susceptible cattle infested with *R. microplus* (Carvalho et al., 2010b), susceptible hosts had an increased blood clotting time at tick hemorrhagic feeding pools in comparison to normal skin and the skin of resistant hosts.

Furthermore, the host resistant phenotype affects the transcript of genes associated with anti-hemostatic proteins in the salivary glands of *R. microplus*, with transcripts coding for anti-coagulant proteins expressed at a higher level in ticks fed on susceptible hosts compared to ticks fed on resistant hosts (Carvalho et al., 2010b).

In the same experiment where PBL gene expression was studied in infested indicine and taurine cattle, the authors examined the response to infestation and larval attachment in bovine skin (Piper et al., 2010).

The susceptible cattle displayed an intense cellular inflammatory response at the tick attachment site, i.e., genes involved in inflammatory processes and immune responses including those which encode for matrix proteins were up-regulated in tick-infested susceptible cattle, but not in resistant hosts.

Nascimento et al. (2010) constructed cDNA libraries from skin biopsies from resistant and susceptible cattle to evaluate the pattern of gene expression of three calcium-binding-proteins. The results showed that genes coding for translationally controlled tumor protein (*1-TPT1*), calcium channel protein transient receptor potential vanilloid 6 (*TRPV6*) and cysteine proteinase inhibitor (*CST6*) were highly expressed in susceptible cattle compared to resistant cattle (Nascimento et al., 2010).

Also, a microarray study using samples from tick infested cattle to evaluate the profile of gene expression during *R. microplus* larvae attachment showed differentially expressed genes involved in lipid metabolism, inflammation control and impairment of tick infestation in resistant cattle (*B. t. indicus* Nelore) (Carvalho et al., 2014).

Conversely, in susceptible cattle (*B. t. taurus* Holstein) the acute phase response appeared impaired but this study confirmed the up-regulation of calcium ion control genes which correlates with the calcium binding proteins reported by Nascimento et al. (2010).

Franzin et al. (2017) also report the up-regulation of protein S100G, another calcium binding protein, in susceptible cattle. An earlier qPCR study showed higher up-regulation of calcium signaling genes in a tick resistant composite breed in response to ticks most predominantly at 24 h post-infestation with larvae (Belmont Red) (Bagnall et al., 2009).

Calcium signaling, calcium binding and/or calcium ion control genes and their functions in tick resistant and tick susceptible cattle warrant further specific examination.

Another host gene expression study was reported recently demonstrating that resistant cattle (*B. t. indicus* Nelore breed) up-regulated the expression of fewer genes encoding enzymes producing volatile compounds that render them less "attractive" to ticks compared with susceptible cattle (*B. t. taurus* Holstein breed) (Franzin et al., 2017).

This finding is consistent with the theory associated with odor (Osterkamp et al., 1999) described above. The study also reported that resistant hosts when exposed to ticks mount an earlier inflammatory response than susceptible cattle (gene expression studies undertaken at 2 days post larval infestation using tick naïve cattle) (Franzin et al., 2017) which appears to disappear later (feeding nymphs at 9 days) but lingers in susceptible cattle.

Franzin et al. (2017) identified numerous novel immune response genes that were up-regulated in susceptible Holstein cattle including *FCER1A* the high affinity immunoglobulin epsilon receptor subunit alpha precursor which is known to be responsible for initiating an allergic response.

The up-regulation of complement *C1QTNF7* (C1q tumor necrosis factor-related protein 7 precursor), an inducer of pro-inflammatory activators (Kishore et al., 2004) also concurs with the conclusions of tick susceptible cattle responding in a pro-inflammatory manner (Piper et al., 2010).

Piper et al. (2008) had identified the up-regulation of Toll-like receptors (i.e., *NFkB*, nuclear factor kappa-light-chain-enhancer of activated B cells) that correlates with the activity of the complement C1Q identified by Franzin et al. (2017).

In addition, *BCL10* (B-cell CLL/lymphoma 10) was up-regulated in susceptible cattle (Franzin et al., 2017) and is also known to activate *NFkB* (Wang M. et al., 2007). In addition fibroleukin is known to have a dual prothrombinase and immunoregulatory activity and was up-regulated in tick naïve (tick susceptible) cattle by larvae (Franzin et al., 2017).

Immunoregulatory activity includes the suppression of T cell proliferation and cytokine production, mainly of Th1 and Th17 cells but not Th2 cells (Bézie et al., 2015), which is in contrast to other observations above suggesting that susceptible cattle mount a Th1 response. Functionally, Bézie et al. (2015) found that fibroleukin induced long-term allograft survival in a rat model through regulatory B cells which in turn suppress the proliferation of CD4+T cells. These cells are up-regulated in tick resistant cattle in the majority of studies undertaken. To summarize the results presented by Franzin et al. (2017), early responses to larvae (48 h post-infestation by naïve tick susceptible cattle) appear to show a mixed Th1 and Th2 response with tick susceptibility being associated with a Th1 response.

Several differences are noted among the comparisons of gene expression studies and as noted by Regitano et al. (2008) we generally concur that "*differences in gene expression of resistant cows compared to susceptible cows were breed-specific.*" However, there are some consistencies identified in the above studies.

The presence of high densities of CD4+, CD25+, and γδ T cells are seen relatively consistently in resistant indicine cattle.

The up-regulation of keratins and collagens is also common in resistant indicine cattle, with some divergent upregulation in susceptible breeds in fewer studies. The up-regulation of IgGs in susceptible cattle was reported by most researchers. MHC Class II and calcium binding proteins seem to be mostly up-regulated in susceptible breeds, with the latter commonly associated with susceptible breeds studied in Brazil. The expression of chemokine ligands varied greatly between studies and breeds with no identifiable consistency.

Other genes that were up-regulated consistently in susceptible cattle include: apolipoproteins (lipid transport), lysozymes (anti-microbial, also found in macrophages and polymorphonuclear neutrophils), Toll like receptors, *NFkB* and NFkB activators *C1QTNF7* (complement C1q tumor necrosis factor –related protein 7) and *BCL10* (B-cell CLL/lymphoma 10) and several complement factors. IL10 is considered an anti-inflammatory cytokine perhaps induced early in susceptible cattle but IL10 appears to be associated with long term resistance in *B. t. indicus* Gyr cattle in Brazil (Domingues et al., 2014; Franzin et al., 2017).

Cytochrome P450 enzymes are a superfamily of hemoproteins known to be involved in the synthesis or metabolism of various molecules and chemicals within cells. A P450 gene called CYP4F3 (cytochrome 450 group 4, subfamily F, gene 3) is known to degrade leukotrienes which are the chemical mediators of allergic responses (Karasuyama et al., 2011).

CYP4F3 was downregulated in the skin of tick exposed resistant cattle (Brahmans, Piper et al., 2010) yet up-regulated in the skin of susceptible cattle (Holsteins, Carvalho et al., 2014) thus showing a correlation for the activity of this enzyme in tick susceptible cattle.

Differential expression of genes coding for other host modifying enzymes were associated with resistant and susceptible phenotypes.

Although not identified in more than one study, the up-regulation of these factors appears to correlate to the relevant phenotype and are thus worthy of further description. For example the following were identified in different studies as up-regulated in tick resistant breeds: Cathepsin B (Wang Y. H. et al., 2007), Cathepsin L2 precursor (cysteine proteases, mast cell mediators) (Nascimento et al., 2011), Cathepsin D (aspartyl protease, mast cell mediator) (Franzin et al., 2017), serine peptidase inhibitor clade A (inhibits neutrophil elastase), phospholipase A2, group VII (platelet activating factor) (Piper et al., 2010), coagulation factors, and procollagen C-endopeptidase enhancer (metalloprotease inhibitor) (Piper et al., 2010); and conversely in tick susceptible breeds: serine peptidase inhibitor clade F (negative regulation of inflammatory response), spleen trypsin inhibitor, plasminogen activator (serine protease which produces plasmin which catalyzes the degradation of fibrin polymers in blood clots), prostaglandin D2 synthase (platelet aggregation inhibitor) (Piper et al., 2010), and phosphoprotein 24 (endopeptidase associated with platelet degranulation) (Franzin et al., 2017) were up-regulated.

Comparative transcriptomic studies of different life stages (larvae and adult females) have shown that ticks respond differentially according to whether they are sensing or feeding on a tick-susceptible or tick-resistant breed of cattle.

A microarray study based on a *R. microplus* EST database (Wang M. et al., 2007), using sensing larvae (not attached to the host but contained within a fabric bag and able to sense the host) and feeding, adult females, which were collected from naïve, tick-susceptible Holstein Friesian *B. t. taurus*, and tick-resistant Brahman *B. t. indicus* cattle has been reported (Rodriguez-Valle et al., 2010).

Ticks that were feeding on resistant cattle demonstrated the up-regulation of serpin 2, lipocalins and histamine binding proteins. A recent study utilized next generation sequencing to compare tick expression differences from larvae, nymph salivary glands and larval offspring of females - all fed on tick-resistant Nelore *B. t. indicus* and tick-susceptible Holstein *B. t. taurus* (Franzin et al., 2017).

That study showed an increased number of transcripts that included evasins, immunosuppressant proteins, lipocalins (including histamine, serotonin, and odorant binding proteins), and reprolysin metalloproteases from ticks associated with susceptible cattle, and an increased number of chitinases and cysteine proteases from ticks associated with resistant cattle. The analysis also included larvae exposed to volatile compounds prepared from the same breeds of cattle and showed that resistant breeds produce less attractive volatiles (Franzin et al., 2017).

The latter was thought to be correlated to the fact that ticks on susceptible cattle up-regulated odorant binding proteins.

Not enough studies have been undertaken to draw any similarities between the molecular profiles of ticks from susceptible vs. resistant hosts particularly when different stages and breeds are compared. It is clear however that the tick gene expression profiles associated with tick-resistant vs. tick-susceptible cattle appear to be divergent.

Acquired immunity to tick infestation is established after a period of susceptibility to a primary infestation (Wagland, 1978). As confirmed above, gene expression profiles from tick resistant breeds appear to be congruent with a T-cell mediated response, while susceptible cattle exhibit innate and inflammatory responses with higher levels of tick specific IgG1.

One quite consistent fact is that resistant cattle appear to be primed to respond to ticks with a higher presence of γδ T cells in the skin of tick naïve resistant cattle in comparison to susceptible. A formal meta-analysis of all gene expression studies where the data are in the public domain is theoretically possible but would likely be compromised by variation in the conditions of each of the studies.

Each gene expression comparison study was undertaken using quite different conditions. The variable factors include: environment, season, naïve vs. tick exposed cattle, the use of acaricides post exposure prior to artificial infestations, infestation protocols including frequency and numbers of larvae, and comparative breeds including within breed studies.

Cellular Physiology Associated with Host Resistance

Granulocytes (or polymorphonuclear leukocytes) are white blood cells characterized by the presence of granules in their cytoplasm and which perform different immune functions. They include neutrophils (most abundant), eosinophils, mast cells, and basophils. The inflammatory profile of the host skin contributes to resistance or susceptibility to tick infestation. Marufu et al. (2013) showed that tick susceptibility (*B. t. taurus* Bonsmara cattle) is associated with an immediate type hypersensitivity reaction.

On the other hand, the resistance phenotype was linked to a delayed hypersensitivity reaction in *B. t. indicus* Nguni breed (Marufu et al., 2013) confirming the observations of Constantinoiu et al. (2010) with *B.t.taurus* Holstein Friesian (susceptible) and *B.t.indicus* Brahman (resistant) cattle.

Neutrophils are usually found in the blood stream and are the most abundant phagocyte. During host infection, neutrophils are quickly recruited to the site of infection i.e., skin in response to tick infestation. Neutrophils may favor infestation by destroying the extracellular matrix around the attached tick and thereby allowing access to blood for feeding (Tatchell and Bennett, 1969; Tatchell and Moorhouse, 1970).

Similar numbers of neutrophils were found to be recruited in Holstein (susceptible, *B. t. taurus*) and Nelore cattle (resistant, *B. t. indicus*) (Carvalho et al., 2010a), with slightly higher neutrophils in the skin of susceptible cattle at early stages of infestation using naïve cattle of the same breeds (Franzin et al., 2017).

Marufu et al. (2014) showed higher counts of neutrophils at the attachment sites of *R. microplus* in both resistant and susceptible breeds compared to non-infested skin, with higher counts also found in tick susceptible Bonsmara cattle compared to tick resistant Nguni cattle (Marufu et al., 2014).

Higher levels of neutrophils do not seem to show a protective role against *R. microplus* infestation and feeding larvae demonstrated a high ingestion of neutrophils in susceptible *B. t. taurus* Holstein Friesian cattle (Constantinoiu et al., 2010).

Moreover, activated neutrophils lead to a calcium ion influx which could correlate with the common up-regulation of calcium binding proteins in susceptible cattle gene expression studies.

Overall, higher neutrophil densities in the skin at the site of a tick attachment appear to be associated with the tick susceptible phenotype.

Eosinophils have long been known to be associated with parasite infections and allergy, with several immune functions having been only recently elucidated.

For example, recent evidence suggests that eosinophils suppress Th17 and Th1 responses via dendritic cell regulation and also activate basophil degranulation (Wen and Rothenberg, 2016).

Eosinophils may influence the tick resistant phenotype due to their role in the translocation of mast cell histamine and lysosomal enzymes to the feeding site lesion, and by impairing tick attachment (Schleger et al., 1981). *B. t. taurus* show higher eosinophil counts during secondary infestations compared with *B. t. indicus* breeds in early studies (Tatchell and Moorhouse, 1968).

Marufu et al. (2013) confirmed this observation with higher eosinophil counts in tick susceptible Bonsmara cattle, in contrast to other studies which showed higher eosinophil counts in tick resistant cattle (Nelore *B. t. indicus*) in Brazil and Australian Shorthorn breed (*B. t.*

taurus tropically adapted cattle) (Schleger et al., 1976; Carvalho et al., 2010b).

Using the same breeds as Carvalho et al. (2010b), Franzin et al. (2017) showed higher eosinophil counts in susceptible cattle during the first infestation of tick naïve cattle, yet higher eosinophil counts at nymph feeding sites in the tick resistant breed. Suppression of Th1 responses by eosinophils may be logically associated with the response of resistant cattle and may also correlate with mast cell activity.

Mast cells (including tissue basophils) are a multifunctional cell population involved in maintaining local homeostasis of connective tissue, control of blood coagulation and defensive functions of innate and adaptive immunity. In addition mast cell dysfunction is associated with several chronic allergic/inflammatory disorders (da Silva et al., 2014).

Mast cells contain granules rich in histamine and heparin, and are the main effectors of allergic reactions. Host resistance to ticks appears to concur with mast cell functions such as allergic responses, wound healing and immune tolerance, and a potential mast cell dysfunction in tick-susceptible cattle.

However, one study comparing several breeds found that the Nelore *B. t. indicus* resistant breed had the highest number of mast cells in response to ticks while the Gyr *B. t. indicus* tick resistant breed had similar levels as two tick susceptible *B. t. taurus* breeds, Holstein and Brown Swiss (Veríssimo et al., 2008).

In contrast, previously Gyr *B. t. indicus* cattle showed a higher number of mast cells in the dermis compared to susceptible European breeds (Moraes et al., 1992; Veríssimo et al., 2008). A few mast cell activators (da Silva et al., 2014) have been noted in resistant host gene expression studies above including Cathepsins B, D, and L2, platelet activating factors, complement factor C3, IL10, IL2, and TNFα.

Basophils are known for their allergic effector function and were first described in response to ticks by Trager in 1939. Basophils notably accumulated at tick bite sites causing cutaneous hypersensitivity (Trager, 1939).

In the 1950s, it was confirmed that histamines are stored in basophil granules (Graham et al., 1955). Basophils have been associated with immunity against parasites including ticks and helminths, reviewed by Karasuyama et al. (2011). It is thus logical as described above for mast cells, that high levels of circulating basophils would be associated with the tick resistant phenotype, which has been confirmed by two groups (Carvalho et al., 2010a; Marufu et al., 2014; Franzin et al., 2017).

The release of histamine has been postulated as a mechanism which dislodges feeding ticks. This was confirmed when mice were injected with cultured mast cells which resulted in tick rejection following infestation of *Haemophysalis longicornis* ticks, with no tick rejection in mast cell deficient mice (Matsuda et al., 1987).

A recent review of basophil functions confirms their effector role in allergic reactions, however basophils also share features of innate and adaptive immunity (Steiner et al., 2016) which again associates well with the tick resistant bovine phenotype. Steiner et al. (2016) examined the ever expanding function of basophils including the modulation of several cytokines, Toll-like receptors and chemokines (including CXCL10, CCR1, CCR7 described as up-regulated.

The correlation of granulocyte activity (and their immune effector mechanisms) in the skin of tick resistant cattle could further be examined to attempt to correlate immunity with gene expression studies described above. The existence of tick histamine-binding salivary lipocalins have been associated with inhibiting histamines from their receptors (Paesen et al., 1999; Mans et al., 2008) with specific lipocalins up-regulated in resistant vs. susceptible breeds in response to ticks (Rodriguez-Valle et al., 2013).

In addition, the central role of histamine in tick resistance was supported by antihistamine administration to cattle which led to increased tick loads on both *B. t. taurus* (Hereford) and *B. t. indicus* (Brahman) breeds (Tatchell and Bennett, 1969).

In summary, these studies confirm that cattle breeds behave differently during *R. microplus* infestation, presenting various intrinsic mechanisms to provide protection against ticks. Overall, resistant cattle appear to be associated with increased mast cells, eosinophils, and basophils in the skin, while the recruitment of neutrophils is potentially associated with tick susceptibility. The release of histamines from these cells appears to be associated with the resistant phenotype.

Histamine is thought to inhibit tick attachment and leads to itching, which subsequently leads to more grooming and tick removal.

Microbiota Role in Tick Resistance

The microbiome contributes to the architecture and function of tissues, host energy metabolism, and also plays an important role in the balance between health and disease as demonstrated recently for intracellular protozoa (Yilmaz et al., 2014; Bär et al., 2015).

In vertebrates, semiochemicals can be generated by the activity of the microbiota upon amino acids, short chain fatty acids or hormones secreted in body emissions, such as sweat, tears, sebum, saliva, breath, urine, and feces (Amann et al., 2014; Fischer et al., 2015).

This volatile repertoire is of paramount importance with evidence that they can direct host-vector specificity (Smallegange et al., 2011; Davis et al., 2013).

The variation in the host chemical production thus causes differential attractiveness to vectors between species and in turn, the bacterial profiles differ according to human genetic background (Benson et al., 2010; Prokop-Prigge et al., 2015).

Microbial composition can be affected by diet and other management strategies, such as those used for beef and dairy cattle (Durso et al., 2012; Thoetkiattikul et al., 2013).

The differences in the composition of their microbiota (Dowd et al., 2008; Durso et al., 2010, 2012; de Oliveira et al., 2013; Mao et al., 2015), as well as the distinct volatile organic compounds (VOC) produced by *B. t. taurus* and *B. t. indicus* cattle may corroborate the contrasting tick infestation phenotypes observed among these animals (Steullet and Gnerin, 1994; Osterkamp et al., 1999; Borges et al., 2015; Ferreira et al., 2015).

Although a few studies have demonstrated that host VOCs play a role in attracting *Rhipicephalus* spp. ticks (Louly et al., 2010; Borges et al., 2015; de Oliveira Filho et al., 2016; Franzin et al., 2017)

DAMAGES CAUSED BY TICKS AND THEIR CONTROL

Ticks comprise veterinary problem because they transmit diseases, produce paralysis or toxicosis, and cause physical damage to livestock. Ticks' species are grouped into three families, Argasidae or soft ticks, Ixodidae or hard ticks and Nuttalliellidae (Klompen et al., 1996).

Ticks are very important to man and his domestic animals, and must be controlled if livestock production is to meet world needs for animal protein. Knowledge of the nature and habits of the tick and the disease agents it transmit helps in control (Stewart et al., 1981).

Losses and control

A complex of problems related to ticks and tick-borne diseases of cattle created a demand for methods to control ticks and reduce losses of cattle (George et al., 2004).

Control of tick infestations and the transmission of tick-borne diseases remain a challenge for the cattle industry in tropical and subtropical areas of the world. Tick control is a priority for many countries in tropical and subtropical regions (Lodos et al., 2000).

Losses due to tick infestations can be considerable. In Australia alone in 1974, losses due to cattle tick (*Boophilus microplus*) were estimated to be USD 62 million (Springell, 1983).

Brazil loses around USD 2 billion per year (Grisi et al., 2002). Such losses can be cut considerably by adopting effective tick control measures.

There are three major reasons for controlling ticks in domestic animals: disease transmission, tick paralysis or toxicosis, and tick-caused physical damage. The main weapon for controlling ticks at present is the use of chemical acaricides (Drummond, 1983).

Ticks are responsible for severe economic losses both through direct effect of blood sucking and indirectly as vector of pathogens and toxins.

1. Direct effect

Feeding by large numbers of ticks causes reduction in live weight and anemia among domestic animals, while tick bites also reduce the quality of hides. Apart from irritation or anemia in case of heavy infestations, tick can cause severe dermatitis (FAO, 1998).

These parasites generate direct effects in cattle in terms of milk production and reduce weight gain (L'Hostis and Seegers, 2002; Peter et al., 2005).

(1) Tick-bite paralysis

It is characterized by an acute ascending flaccid motor paralysis caused by the injection of a toxin by certain ticks while feeding. Examples are paralysis caused by the feeding of *Dermacentor andersoni*, sweating sickness caused by *Hyalomma truncatum*, Australian tick paralysis caused by *Ixodes holocylus*, and tick toxicosis caused by *Rhipicephalus* species (Drummond, 1983).

Tick paralysis is most common in late winter and spring when the adult ticks are active, but it can occur at any time if the weather is warm and humid (Stewart and de Vos, 1984).

Paralysis in cattle caused by *Ixodes holocyclus* and *Dermacentor andersoni* had also been reported by Doube and Kemp (1975) and Lysyk et al.(2005) respectively.

(2) Physical damage

Ticks are attached to the body for a blood meal and may cause irritation and serious physical damages to livestock. Included are "tick worry", irritation, unrest, and weight loss due to massive infestation of ticks; the direct injury to hides due to tick bites, loss of blood due to the feeding of ticks (Drummond, 1983).

2. Vector of pathogens

Ticks can be carrier, of pathogens, which they transmit from host to host during blood sucking and cause a large variety of diseases (FAO, 1998).

The major diseases include Babesiosis, Anaplasmosis, Theileriosis, and heart-water, East Coast fever; in addition, other diseases of lesser importance cause severe economic losses to the livestock industry (Drummond, 1983; Bram, 1983).

The presence, dynamics and amount of parasite stock in ticks exert a major influence on the kinetics of transmission of tick-borne parasitic diseases (Morel, 1980).

Generally the ticks become infested with the causative organisms of diseases while they are feeding on infected animals. Then the organism may be transmitted from stage to stage in the tick (an example is *Theileria parva* transmitted by *Rhipicephalus appendiculatus*), or from the female tick through the egg to the larvae—an increase of several thousand times in vector potential (an example is *Babesia equi* transmitted by Anocentor nitens). When the next stage or generation subsequently feeds on another animal, the organism is transmitted to that animal if it is susceptible to the disease (Drummond, 1983).

Tick born diseases generally affect the blood and/or lymphatic system (FAO, 1998). Tick fever organisms, like *Anaplasma marginale*, are significant causes of cattle morbidity in Australia, USA, China and other countries (CRC-VT, 2001).

Cattle tick *B. microplus*, economically impact cattle production by transmitting pathogens that cause Babesiosis (*B. bovis* and *B. bigemina*) and Anaplasmosis (*A. marginale*) (Peter et al., 2005).

Chemical control of ticks

There are several methods being applied for controlling ticks and tick-borne diseases. The main weapon for the control of ticks at present is the use of chemical acaricides. Acaricides used to control ticks on livestock or in the environment are applied in such a manner that the ticks are killed, but will not harm livestock or applicators, the tissues of treated animals will not contain chemical residues, and the environment will not be adversely affected (Drummond, 1983).

The conventional control methods include the use of chemical acaricides with partially successful results but this treatment has certain implicit drawbacks, such as the presence of residues in the milk and meat and the development of chemical resistant tick strains (Willadsen and Kemp, 1988; Nolan, 1990).

The use of acaricides has disadvantages, such as the selection of resistant tick populations and harmful effects on the animals, human beings and the environment (García-García et al., 2000).

The development of new acaricides is a long and expensive process, which reinforces the need for alternative approaches to control tick infestations (Graf et al., 2004).

Certain herbal mixtures with 70% efficacy for tick control have also been reported by Regassa (2000).

1. Acaricides

Control of tick infestation through the use of acaricides is one of the methods that can be used to reduce the tick-borne diseases (Spickett and Fivaz, 1992).

A wide range of acaricides, including arsenical, chlorinated hydrocarbons, organophosphates, carbamates and synthetic pyrethroids are being used for controlling ticks on livestock. The performance of an acaricide in the control of ticks depends not only on the activity of a product, but on the quality and quantity of active ingredient deposited on cattle or delivered internally (George, 2000).

2. Arsenic

Use of arsenic was the first effective method for controlling ticks and tick-borne diseases, and was used in many parts of the world before resistance to the chemical became a problem (George, 2000).

It was first used for tick control in 1893 in South Africa (Bekker, 1960) that is inexpensive, stable, and water soluble, and there is an accurate vat-side test (Drummond, 1983).

Arsenic was the first acaricides to be widely used which is cheapest and most effective agent. Mostly it is used in the form of water soluble compounds like sodium arsenite. Usually As_2O_3 have been used for many years in dipping vats to control ticks, especially ticks of the genus *Boophilus*. Arsenic dips were used successfully to eradicate *Boophilus* ticks from the southern United States. Unfortunately, arsenic has a very short residual effectiveness (less than one to two days), and in most areas of the world *Boophilus* ticks have become resistant to arsenic (Drummond, 1983).

3. Chlorinated hydrocarbons

These are synthetic acaricides. Resistance to arsenicals was developed in many species of ticks (Matthewson and Baker, 1975; Angus, 1996) and it was replaced by chlorinated hydrocarbons (Graham and Hourrigan, 1977).

Chlorinated hydrocarbon acaricides are very persistent and have been used extensively throughout the world for controlling ticks. Of particular interest are benzene hexachloride toxaophene (Drummond, 1983).

Their mode of action is by interfering with nerve conduction of ticks (Solomon, 1983). Because of their high toxicity and long lifespan, these compounds have mostly been withdrawn from the market (Spickett, 1998).

4. Organophosphorous compounds

Organophosphates were introduced around 1950, as a replacement for the chlorinated hydrocarbons to which significant resistance had occurred (Shanahan and Hart, 1966).

These are esters of phosphoric acid and have a wide range of activities against ticks at very low concentration in companion and livestock animals. However, their residual effectiveness is usually shorter than that of chlorinated hydrocarbons, and the risk of causing acute toxicity in livestock is greater (Drummond, 1983).

Resistance in ticks was first recognized in 1963 and several tick species are now known to be resistant to organophosphorous acaricides (Wharton, 1967).

5. Carbamates

These are esters of carbamic acids and closely resemble the organophosphates (Spickett, 1998). They are a little more toxic than the organophosphates for mammals and are much more expensive.

Application of chemicals

Various methods including dipping, spraying, ear tagging or pour on, have been used to apply chemicals to protect livestock against ticks. Direct application of acaricides to animals is the most popular method of controlling ticks on livestock (Drummond, 1983).

Applications of acaricide to tick-infested cattle via dipping or sprayer can be equally effective under ideal conditions with proper handling of equipments without injuring animals and subsequent dilution of a product (George, 2000).

1. Dipping

In this method, animals are immersed in a dipping tub containing solution of chemicals. By 1893 in Australia, Africa, and the United States the use of "dipping-vats" to immerse tick-infested cattle in a variety of chemical agents was a component of the effort to control the ticks and tick-borne diseases affecting cattle (Mohler, 1906; Matthewson and Baker, 1975).

A variety of tickicides including cottonseed oil, fish oil, crude petroleum, kerosene, creosote, tobacco extract, soap, and a combination of sulphur and kerosene were among the hundreds of possible acaricides tested for dipping (Mohler, 1906; Angus, 1996).

Infested cattle should be dipped in the organophosphate acaricide coumaphos (0.3% active ingredient) (Bram et al., 2002). In general, dipping vats provide a highly effective method of treating animals with acaricides for tick control. However, their immobility, high initial cost of construction, and the cost of the acaricides may make vats impractical for many small ranching operations.

Also, dipping vats must be managed carefully so that the dips are maintained at the proper concentration and the cattle are dipped properly (Drummond, 1983).

2. Spray

The application of fluid acaricides to an animal by means of a spray has many advantages and has been successfully practiced for controlling ticks on most of the animals (Barnett, 1961).

Spraying equipment is highly portable, and only small amounts of acaricides need to be mixed for a single application. However, spraying is generally less efficient in controlling ticks than immersion in a dipping vat because of problems associated with applying the acaricides thoroughly on all parts of the animal body (Drummond, 1983).

3. Spot treatment or hand dressing

There are predilections sites for certain tick species on part of the body which are not effectively treated by spray or dips. The inner parts of the ear, under part of the tail, the tail brush and the areas between the teats and the legs in cattle with large udder, are especially liable to escape treatment. Acaricides may be applied to these sites by hand is termed as hand dressing (Barnett, 1961) or spot treatment.

The application of insecticides with aerosols and in oils, smears, and dusts by hand to limited body areas is time-consuming and laborious, but in certain instances it may be more effective and economical (in terms of cost of acaricide) than treating the entire animal (Drummond, 1983).

4. Some other applications

Some other methods of applying acaricides are ear tags, neck bands, tail bands and pour-one, particularly for the pyrethroids with long residual activity. A mechanical applicator was also developed (Duncan, 1991).

In Kenya, an intraruminal ivermectin slow-release device provided 90 d protection against tick damage (Tatchell, 1992). Tick repellents used on livestock are limited (Mwase et al., 1990).

Ivermectin has been delivered orally in the case of *Boophilus annulatus* on cattle by Millar et al.(2001) as a single or double ruminal bolus as daily capsules to *B. miroplus* infested cattle. The control levels against standard engorging female ticks reached 99%. Despite this, the level of control of ticks on pastures grazed by treated cattle was insufficient to prevent cattle from becoming infested when grazed there later on.

Abdel-Shafy and Zayed (2002) examined the acaricidal effect of plant extract of neem seed oil (*Azadirachta indica*) on egg, immature and adult stages of *Hyalomma anatolicum excavatum*. This short communication on the potential use of azadirachtin for tick control is an extension from the large volume of literature on this material for control of crop pests and vectors of medical pathogens.

Azadirachtin was applied at concentrations of 1.6% through to 12.8% in water and applied to ticks in vitro for 1 min. The ticks were examined up to 15 d post treatment for mortality and reduced viability.

Abdel-Shafy and Zayed (2002) concluded that Neem can be used for tick control at economic concentrations of 1.6% to 3.2%. The work will need to be enlarged to test control of feeding ticks on cattle and possibly control of ticks by spraying the moulting and resting site of ticks in cattle pens.

Safety measures

Appropriate directions and precautions given on the label, should be taken while applying the acaricides. According to U.S. Department of Agriculture (1967), these acaricides can be toxic to livestock and humans, can create residues in tissues of animals, and may be destructive to the environment if they are not used and handled in a safe and correct manner. The safe use of acaricides is essential to an efficient, well-run program for control of ticks.

To avoid accidents and misuse, it is necessary to continually review and employ safe use, precautions and procedures (Drummond, 1983). It is important to prepare dipping and spray fluids correctly to ensure that a dose of the active ingredient, lethal for the tick, is administered to cattle safely and without exceeding the limits for milk and meat residues.

Licking behavior and environmental contamination arising from pour-on ivermectin for cattle was studied by Laffont et al.(2001) and was found to be associated with unexpected residues in meat and dairy products and as an environmental contaminant via cattle dung. They recommended that the route of potential contamination of parasiticides be taken into account during product registration.

RESISTANCE

Tick resistance to acaricides is an increasing problem and real economic threat to the livestock and allied industries. Most stock holders depend completely on acaricides to control ticks, but do not have access to guidelines on how to make a profit from their tick control program or how to detect and resolve problems with resistance to acaricides (George, 2000).

Resistance has led to instability and increased costs in areas where the one-host cattle ticks *Boophilus microplus* and *B. decoloratus* have acquired resistance to a variety of toxic chemicals. The point has now been reached where such resistance must be expected in these ticks within five to 10 years of the introduction of any new type of acaricide, unless control practices are changed (Wharton, 1983).

The evolution of tick resistance to acaricides has been a major determinant of the need for new products (George, 2000).

Fernandes (2001) worked on toxicological effects and resistance to pyrethroids in *Boophilus microplus* from Goias, Brazil. According to his research ticks were resistant to deltamethrin and cypermethrin, and showed the required level of mortality only to high concentrations of permethrin.

Considering the frequency with which synthetic pyrethroid resistance has been reported in Brazil, and elsewhere, the claim of resistance is very likely to be correct. Sseruga et al.(2003) studied the serological evidence of exposure to tick fever organisms in young cattle on Queensland dairy farms. They concluded that, in tick-infested areas, vaccination is the most effective means of protecting cattle against tick fever. Resistance detection, identification and characterization of resistance were briefly reviewed by Wharton (1983).

Resistance is usually recognized because of failure to obtain a satisfactory kill of the parasitic stages on treated animals. Failure is frequently due to inadequate treatment and many reports of resistance are unfounded. There is no doubt about resistance when cattle continue to be infested with large numbers of engorged ticks after frequent treatments. But the response of parasitic ticks to under strength acaricides is very similar to their response to low-level resistance or to high-level resistance in the early stages of its development. Thus field-spraying tests must be conducted under standardized conditions where resistance is suspected (Baker and Shaw, 1965).

A survey of cattle tick control practices in South Africa found that 35.7% of farmers using hand sprays have confirmed acaricide resistance compared with 25.8% and 23.9% of users of spray races and plunge-dips respectively (Spickett and Fivaz, 1992).

Confirmation of resistance must be made by laboratory tests. The traditional test for diagnosing resistance to acaricides in single host ticks is the larval packet test, in which larvae are placed in envelopes impregnated with acaricide (Wharton and Roulston, 1970). Mainly chemical companies in screening programmes have developed many methods of testing the effects of acaricides.

The stages most commonly used are the engorged females and the unfed larvae. The former usually provide the most useful information on potential acaricides, but unfed larvae are generally accepted as the logical stage to document resistance. Several engorged females provide sufficient larvae to test against a range of concentrations of several acaricides.

The response of susceptible ticks provides the baseline when resistance is suspected (Wharton, 1983). Resistance in *B. microplus* populations in Australia and South Africa to arsenic was observed about 50 years after use of the chemical began (Matthewson and Baker, 1975; Angus, 1996).

Host resistance

Resistance to tick infestation varies among individuals and breed of cattle. It is known that in many subtropical and semi-arid environments in Africa indigenous dual purpose breeds are highly resistant to ticks, resulting in low infestation rates that cause significant direct losses (Norval et al., 1991).

The phenomena of host resistance to ticks and enzootic stability to tick born diseases are well documented (Perry et al., 1985; Latif and Pegram, 1992).

ALTERNATIVE METHODS OF TICK CONTROL

Due to the present disadvantages of chemical acaricide products, the adoption of alternative methods could minimize such problems. Wharton (1983) briefly reviewed the alternative methods of tick control and concluded that the utilization of host resistance, while offering an attractive approach to tick control, raises many questions even with the relatively simple *B. microplus-Babesia* association.

Resistance is an acquired characteristic and each animal develops its own level of resistance in response to tick challenge; the level may be high (as in most zebu cattle) or low (as in most European cattle), but a wide range of resistance occurs in all breeds of cattle.

It is heritable, and selection and breeding for tick resistance are possible not only in zebu×European breeds, but also within European breeds. However, selection for resistance or culling for susceptibility must at present be based on tick numbers surviving on cattle exposed either naturally or artificially to tick challenge. This raises obvious problems for the cattle producer who is concerned about the effects of these ticks on production. Breeding of tick resistance cattle, pasture spelling, pasture burning and some special grasses have also been considered for tick control.

Bock et al.(1997) compared two breeds of cattle and reported that *Bos indicus* had innate resistance to infection with *babesia bovis*, *B. bigemina* and *Anaplasma marginale* as compared to *Bos taurus* breed.

Wharton (1983) reviewed that the most logical method of alleviating tick depredations would be to capitalize on host-parasite relationships that evolved in nature.

Cattle survived in Asia and Africa despite *Babesia*, *Theileria* and their *Boophilus* and *Rhipicephalus* vectors. Host resistance, expressed by an animal's ability to prevent the maturing of large numbers of ticks, and disease immunity, are survival mechanisms for the host and for external and internal parasites.

The problem is not only to utilize these attributes, but also to increase productivity. Resistance to *B. microplus* is associated primarily with zebu (*Bos indicus*) cattle. Considerable progress has been made in evolving resistant *Bos indicus*×*Bos taurus* beef and dairy cattle that limit the effects of ticks while retaining high productivity (Turner, 1975; Hayman, 1974; Mason, 1974).

Pasture spelling, pasture burning and use of certain grasses and legumes are also practiced for inhibition or killing of ticks (Branagan, 1973; Sutherst et al., 1982; Chiera et al., 1984).

Improvement of the nutrient value of pasture would allow cattle to develop a better resistance to tick infestation (Sutherst, 1983). Gladney et al.(1974) concluded that insect control based on sterile males or genetic manipulations offer little promise while pheromone attractants could be useful for domestic pets, or for ticks attached on specialized sites. Mbati et al.(2002) reported that farmers also used alternative methods such as used engine oil (12%), Jeyes fluid (24%), chickens (4%) and de-ticking (2%).

Kaaya and Hassan (2000) reported that the use of entomopathogenic fungi to control ticks may reduce the frequency of chemical acaricide use and the need for treatment for tick-borne diseases. They also conclude that mycopesticides are safer for the environment than conventional acaricides.

Immunological control through vaccines

Several approaches have been used to actively immunize bovines against the cattle tick. The first attempts included the use of complex tick extracts (Willadsen et al., 1988).

For both, ticks and tick-borne diseases, vaccines have been developed or are in the course of being developed. Although tick-borne diseases are important in all domestic animals, vaccine development and production has so far focused on the economically important tick-borne diseases of cattle, such as Babesiosis (*B. bovis*, *B. bigemina*), Theileriosis (*T. parva*, *T. annulata*), Anaplasmosis (*A. marginale*) and Cowdriosis (*C. ruminantium*).

FAO has been implementing a coordinated multi-donor programme for integrated tick and tick-borne disease control in Eastern, Central and Southern Africa. Vaccine development, production and delivery were the main focus of that programme.

A three strain *Theileria parva* stabilize vaccine, known as the Muguga cocktail was developed. This vaccine has been used in combination with an antibiotic treatment, known as the infection-and-treatment method.

Later the mild Boleni strain was isolated for vaccine production in Zimbabwe and is currently being used without the treatment component (FAO, 1998). Scientists are working towards new and improved vaccine of tick fever to replace existing one. Existing vaccines have a high level of side effects, low coverage and can be expensive to make (CRC-VT, 2001).

Willadsen (2001) worked on the molecular revolution in the development of vaccines against ecto-parasites. He warns that there is a long way to go before the full potential of anti-tick vaccines will be reached and they will very likely need to be multiple antigen formulation. However, he and his coworkers pioneering work on the Bm86 based vaccines remain the best example of a commercial recombinant vaccine in the tick and tick-borne pathogens field.

The recombinant Bm86-containing vaccine against the cattle tick *Boophilus microplus* has proved its efficacy in a number of experiments, especially when combined with acaricides in an integrated manner (García-García et al., 2000).

Tellam et al.(2002) studied the reduced oviposition of *Boophilus microplus* feeding on sheep vaccinated vitelline. He used both vitelline and the protein GP80 with which it has immunological cross reactivity. Two vaccines against the tick *Boophilus microplus* have been developed. They are being field tested in Brazil in collaboration with FAO. Although there is a vaccine available, their efficiency is not 100%, which is why there is need to have an improved and absolute vaccine that can help cure animal stock against ticks (FAO, 1998).

Jenkins (2001) studied "Advances and prospects for subunit vaccines against protozoa of veterinary importance". Tick-borne diseases in his review were Babesiosis and Theileriosis. Because of the risk associated with using live parasites (such as the need for a cold chain, limited shelf-life, clinical reactions, reversion of attenuation), research towards subunit vaccines is rapidly advancing.

But their development is complicated by several factors, such as antigenic variation and strain diversity. The generation of a protective immune response furthermore depends on other factors, for instance delivery, adjutant, age of the animal, etc. The identification of protective tick antigens remains a major limitation in the development of further anti-tick vaccines as well as a significant scientific challenge.

García-García et al.(2000) reported the isolation of the Bm95 gene from the *B. microplus* strain A, and found that Bm95 antigen from strain A was able to protect against infestations with Bm86-sensitive and Bm86-resistant tick strains.

He suggested that Bm95 could be a more universal antigen to protect cattle against infestations by *B. microplus* strains from different geographical areas. Almazán et al.(2003) conducted research on identification of protective antigens for the control of *Ixodes scapularis* infestation using cDNA expression library immunization.

Chemical Control

Control of ticks with acaricides may be directed against the free-living stages in the environment or against the parasitic stages on hosts. Control of ixodid ticks by acaricide treatment of vegetation has been done in specific sites (eg, along trails) in recreational areas in the USA and elsewhere, to reduce the risk of tick attachment to people.

This method has not been recommended for wider use because of environmental pollution and the cost of treatment of large areas. Dog kennels, barns, and human dwellings may also require periodic treatment with acaricides to control the free-living stages of ixodid ticks such as the kennel tick, *Rhipicephalus sanguineus*.

The free-living stages of argasid ticks, which infest specific foci such as fowl runs, pigeon lofts, pig sties, and human dwellings, are more frequently and more effectively treated with acaricides.

Treatment of hosts with acaricides to kill attached larvae, nymphs, and adults of ixodid ticks and larvae of argasid ticks has been the most widely used control method. A variety of ectoparasiticide products are available on the market to treat animals against ticks.

Some ectoparasiticides are applied as sprays, dips/washes, spot-on treatments, or impregnated tugs and collars and distributed cutaneously—on the skin surface. Others are administered orally and distributed systemically by the blood circulation. In general, ticks must attach to an animal and acquire a blood meal for the blood-distributed ectoparasiticides to be effective. Alternatively, cutaneously distributed ectoparasiticides have a potential to both kill the attached ticks and prevent the attachment of new ones.

Pyrethroids, including fipronil, permethrin, and permethrin combination products, are effective ectoparasiticides because of rapid penetration of arthropod cuticle and high accumulation in arthropod tissues. However, topically applied cutaneous ectoparasiticides may not achieve a uniform distribution, with some body parts not being covered to the same extent and concentration (eg, hind legs vs. the back).

This may be due to the distance from the original application site as well as by greater comparative loss of active ingredient from the legs because of routine life activities.

Pyrethroids are safe and effective in dogs; however, they are toxic to cats and fish. Systemically distributed ectoparasiticides, including afoxolaner, fluralaner, and sarolaner, tend to achieve more uniform distribution throughout the animal body and extremities but may take longer to reach the full efficacy and have somewhat lower speed of kill.

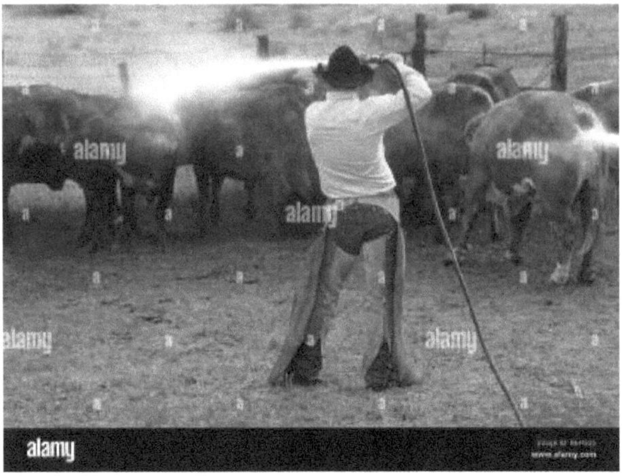

Vaccines

An advance of potentially great importance has been the production, using biotechnology, of a promising vaccine against *R microplus*. The immunizing agent is a concealed tick antigen, not normally encountered by the host.

The immune mechanism it stimulates is different from that stimulated by exposure to ticks (ie, tick feeding). The antigen was derived from a crude extract of partially engorged adult female ticks. It stimulates the production of an antibody that damages tick gut cells and kills the ticks or drastically reduces their reproductive potential.

Prospects of developing similar vaccines against other ixodid tick vectors of cattle diseases of major veterinary importance are not clear. *Rhipicephalus* ticks are good candidates for such vaccines in that they are one-host ticks and show a marked preference for bovine hosts, which act as the principal reservoir of perhaps the most important group of disease agents (*Babesia* spp) these ticks transmit.

By contrast, most other tick vector species of agents that cause important cattle diseases (eg, anaplasmosis, heartwater, theileriosis) are three-host ticks, which infest not only cattle but also wild ungulate species, for which vaccination is not feasible. Moreover, many wild ungulate hosts of the vector ticks serve as reservoirs of these disease agents.

For these reasons, vaccines against nonboophilid vector ticks may be unable either to eradicate the ticks or to eliminate important sources of the disease agents they transmit.

Control Strategies

Initially, the main uses of acaricides were for tick eradication, prevention of spread of ticks and tickborne diseases (quarantine), and eradication and control of tickborne diseases.

The eradication programs were successful in some ecologically marginal subtropical areas, such as southern USA and central Argentina where *Rhipicephalus* spp and babesiosis were eradicated, and southern Africa where East Coast fever (caused by *Theileria parva parva*) was eradicated.

The programs were less successful in the ecologically more favorable tropical areas of northeastern Australia, Central America, the Caribbean Islands, and East Africa.

In the areas where eradication was not achieved, costs of maintaining intensive tick control programs often have become prohibitive. For this reason, integrated biologic and chemical control strategies are being adopted. The effectiveness of these cost-containment strategies requires better knowledge of the dynamic associations among the disease agents, their vertebrate hosts, the tick vectors, and the environment.

Strict quarantine measures to prevent reintroductions are enforced in countries from which ticks and tickborne diseases have been eradicated. Climate-matching models, geographic information systems, and expert systems (models based on expert knowledge and artificial intelligence) are being used to identify unaffected areas in which tick pests could become established if introduced.

Control of these diseases will require use of the principles of endemic stability and development of improved recombinant vaccines. A current, promising strategy is the identification of receptor sites on the midgut of vector ticks and the development of antibodies that bind with these sites, thereby blocking tick-ingested tickborne pathogens from infecting the tick.

Cattle injected with receptor-site antigens may produce antibodies that feeding ticks ingest.

Management of Host Animals

Food and shelter are essential requisites for wildlife. The residential landscape can be particularly attractive to white-tailed deer and conducive to mice and chipmunks, important hosts in the prevalence of ticks and Lyme disease.

One component of a tick management strategy is managing deer and small rodent activity in your yard. Some landscaping practices discussed in the previous section can also help manage key animals in the landscape. Stonewalls, woodpiles, and dense vegetation can harbor rodents.

Host-Targeted Chemical Tick Control for White-tailed deer

The U.S. Department of Agriculture, Agricultural Research Service (ARS), developed passive self-treatment methods for white-tailed deer through both systemic (i.e. ivermectin-treated corn) and topical application technologies to kill ticks feeding on deer.

A device termed a '4-Poster' was designed for the application of topical acaricides to white-tailed deer to prevent the successful feeding of adult ticks. It consists of a feeding station with four paint rollers that hold the pesticide.

Deer self treat themselves when, because of the design, they are forced to brush against the rollers as they feed on whole kernel corn. Computer simulations of various intervention scenariossuggested that acaricide applied to white-tailed deer (assuming 90% of deer are treated and 90% tick mortality on these deer) would prevent more cases of human Lyme disease except perhaps for the best use scenario of a Lyme disease vaccine.

Because white-tailed deer are the keystone species for adult blacklegged ticks and lone star ticks, the '4-Poster' was evaluated on free-ranging deer in a multi-year (5 years treatment plus 2 additional years tick sampling) project in the northeastern United States for the control of both tick species at seven 2-mi2 sites in 5 states (MD, NJ, NY, CT, RI). Approximately one device was placed per 51 acres, although some minimally used 4-posters were redeployed near heavily used devices to increase host access. Treatments utilized a 2% oily formulation of amitraz and reduced blacklegged tick abundance by up to 81% and lone star ticks up to 99.5% in the treated communities in comparison with untreated areas after 3 or more years of use.

Similarly, the application of 10% permethrin to a 600-acre fenced population of deer resulted in a 91-100% reduction of larval, nymphal, and adult questing blacklegged ticks at the Goddard Space Flight Center, MD. While usage of the devices by deer was generally high (> 90 to 100%), utilization of the devices by deer can be low or sporadic when alternative food sources were available such as heavy acorn mast.

Maintenance of the feed and topical insecticide through the tick season is labor intensive. Nevertheless, according to computer simulations, this approach, in principal, could provide the greatest reduction in Lyme disease with the least direct community involvement (i.e. number of direct participating households) and may be an alternative to the application of area-wide acaricides and the maintenance of drastically reduced deer populations.

The '4-Poster' Deer Treatment Bait Station is licensed to the American Lyme Disease Foundation of Lyme, CT (www.aldf.com) and manufactured by C. R. Daniels, Inc. of Ellicott City, MD (www.crdaniels.com). The U.S. Environmental Protection Agency (EPA) has registered an oily 10% permethrin formulation of ready to use tickicide (Y-TEX '4-Poster' Tickicide®, Y-TEX Corporation, Cody, WY) especially for application to deer via the '4-Poster Deer Treatment

Stations to control I. scapularis and A. americanum. Permethrin is the chemical used as a tick repellent on clothing and as an acaricide in some louse and scabies mite treatment products for human use. According to the 'Tickicide' label, the acaricide is not to be used less than 100 yards from any home, apartment, playground, or other place children might be present without adult supervision.

States may impose more restrictive requirements than the federal label. State pesticide registrations have been obtained in 47 of the 48 contiguous states except for New York, which has strict regulations against feeding deer. Approval requirements or regulations for use by state wildlife offi cials vary from state to state and use of the device raises some concerns among some state wildlife agencies. Although no cases have been observed in New England and only a single isolated occurrence in New York, Chronic Wasting Disease (CDW) has been shown to be transmitted via blood and saliva of infected deer, primarily in Michigan and other north central states. The use of the 4-poster will probably be most practical as part of a neighborhood or community coordinated program to reduce ticks and the risk of Lyme disease, managed under state use regulations, and combined with some form of a deer management program.

CONCLUSION

It is concluded that ticks cause great economic losses to livestock in the world and adversely effect livestock host in several ways and parasitized a wide range of vertebrate hosts, and transmit a wider variety of pathogenic agents than any other group of arthropods.

In the area of tick control, much has been achieved, but much more remains to be done. The availability of vaccine is very small. The ability to induce an effective, sustained immunological response is crucial but needs improvement.

Problems of acaricide resistance, chemical residues in food and the environment and the unsuitability of tick resistant cattle for all production systems make the current situation unsatisfactory and require the development of absolute control through effective vaccine.

Taking advantage of recent advances from new approaches and technologies as applied to the field of vector biology, such as transcriptomics, proteomics, immune-molecular characterization, elucidation of naturally acquired resistance, and the development of innovative arthropod and animal models, may lead to improved investigations of naturally acquired resistant breeds against tick and tick-borne pathogens.

Immune-proteomic, sialotranscriptome and reverse genetics/gene editing (RNAi, CRISPR/Cas9) may help to identify new vaccine candidates that resist ticks and tick-borne pathogens. By understanding the tick:host interface and the most common denominators of immunity to ticks, this acquired immune response could be manipulated to improve the efficacy of novel anti-tick vaccines.

Conversely, the knowledge obtained may assist in the selection of tick resistant cattle or the manipulation of susceptible cattle to develop a protective tick immune response. Furthermore, the in depth analysis of host microbiota and volatile organic compounds could lead to probiotic or diet changes or inhibitory chemicals which could render susceptible cattle less attractive to ticks.

Future research may lead to a combination of several of these technologies as novel tick and tick-borne disease control options by first identifying viable biological targets and dissecting pathways leading to vaccination or pharmaceutical therapies or cattle management opportunities for tick control.

REFERENCES

Abbas, R. Z., Zaman, M. A., Colwell, D. D., Gilleard, J., and Iqbal, Z. (2014). Acaricide resistance in cattle ticks and approaches to its management: the state of play. *Vet. Parasitol.* 203, 6–20. doi: 10.1016/j.vetpar.2014.03.006

Abdel-Shafy S, Zayed AA. In vitro acaricidal effect of plant extract of neem seed oil (*Azadirachta indica*) on egg, immature and adult stages of *Hyalomma anatolicum excavatum* (Ixodoidea: Ixodidae) *Vet Parasitol.* 2002;**106**(1):89–96. doi: 10.1016/S0304-4017(02)00023-7.

Ackerman, S., Clare, F. B., McGill, T. W., and Sonenshine, D. E. (1981). Passage of host serum components, including antibody, across the digestive tract of *Dermacentor variabilis* (Say). *J. Parasitol.* 67, 737–740. doi: 10.2307/3280459

Acosta-Rodriguez, R., Alonso-Morales, R., Balladares, S., Flores-Aguilar, H., Garcia-Vazquez, Z., and Gorodezky, C. (2005). Analysis of BoLA class II microsatellites in cattle infested with *Boophilus microplus* ticks: class II is probably associated with susceptibility. *Vet. Parasitol.* 127, 313–321. doi: 10.1016/j.vetpar.2004.10.007

Allen, J. R. (1989). Immunology of interactions between ticks and laboratory animals. *Exp. Appl. Acarol.* 7, 5–13. doi: 10.1007/BF01200448

Allen, J. R., and Humphreys, S. J. (1979). Immunisation of guinea pigs and cattle against ticks. *Nature* 280, 491–493. doi: 10.1038/280491a0

Almazán C, Kocan KM, Bergman DK, García-García JC, Blouin EF, del la Fuente J. Identification of protective antigens for the control of *Ixodes scapularis* infestation using cDNA expression library immunization. *Vaccine.* 2003;**21**(13-14):1492–1501. doi: 10.1016/S0264-410X(02)00683-7.

Amann, A., de Lacy Costello, B., Miekisch, W., Schubert, J., Buszewski, B., Pleil, J., et al. (2014). The human volatilome: volatile organic compounds (VOCs) in exhaled breath, skin emanations, urine, feces and saliva. *J. Breath. Res.* 8:034001. doi: 10.1088/1752-7155/8/3/034001

Angus BM. The history of the cattle tick *Boophilus microplus* in Australia and achievements in its control. *Aust Soc Parasitol.* 1996;**26**:1341–1355.

Antle, J. M, Cole, D. C and Crissman, C. C. 1998. Integrated simulation model and analysis of economic, environmental, and health tradeoffs in the Carchi potatopasture production system. In: Crissman, C. C, Antle, J. M, Capalbo, S. M., Economics, environmental and health tradeoffs in agriculture: Pesticides and the sustainability of Andean potato production, pp.243-266. International Potato Center. Kluwer Academic Publishers. DordrechtIBostonILondon.

Antle, J. M and Pingali, P., 1994. Health and productivity effects of pesticide use in Philippine rice production. Resources, vol. 144, pp. 16-19.

Antle,1. M and Pingali, P., 1994a. Pesticides, productivity, and farmer health: A Philippine case study. American Journal of Agricultrural Economics, voL 76, pp. 418-430.

Antle, J. M and Capalbo, S. M., 1994. Pesticides, productivity, and farmer health: Implications for regulatory policy and agricultural research. American Journal of Agricultrural Economics, vol. 76, pp. 598-602.

Antle, J. M, Cole, D. C, Crissman, C. C., 1998. Further evidence on pesticides, productivity and farmer health: Potato production in Ecuador. Agricultural Economics, vol. 18, pp. 199-207.

Ashton, G. C., Seifert, G. W., and Francis, J. (1968). An association between serum amylase phenotype and tick infestation in cattle. *Aust. J. Biol. Sci.* 21, 303–308.

Bagnall, N., Gough, J., Cadogan, L., Burns, B., and Kongsuwan, K. (2009). Expression of intracellular calcium signalling genes in cattle skin during tick infestation. *Parasite Immunol.* 31, 177–187. doi: 10.1111/j.1365-3024.2008.01092.x

Baker JFA, Shaw RD. Toxaphene and lindane resistance in *Rhipicephalus appendiculatus*, the brown ear tick of equatorial and southern Africa. *J S Afr Vet Med Ass.* 1965;**36**:321–330.

Bär, A.-K., Phukan, N., Pinheiro, J., and Simoes-Barbosa, A. (2015). The interplay of host microbiota and parasitic protozoans at mucosal interfaces: implications for the outcomes of infections and diseases. *PLoS Negl. Trop. Dis.* 9:e0004176. doi: 10.1371/journal.pntd.0004176

Barendse, W. (2007). *Assessing Tick Resistance in a Bovine Animal for Selecting Cattle for Tick Resistance by Providing a Nucleic Acid from the Bovine Animal and Assaying for the Occurrence of a Single Nucleotide Polymorphism (SNP).* Patent No. WO2007051248 A1.

Barker SC, Murrell A. Systematics and evolution of ticks with a list of valid genus and species names. *Parasitology.* 2004;**129**(7):S15–S36. doi: 10.1017/S0031182004005207.

Barré, N., and Uilenberg, G. (2010). Spread of parasites transported with their hosts: case study of two species of cattle tick. *Rev. Sci. Tech.* 29, 149–160. Available online at: https://www.oie.int/doc/ged/D7236.PDF

Barnett SF. *The Control of Ticks on Livestock.* Rome, Italy: Food and Agriculture Organization of the United Nations; 1961. p. 115. Agriculture Studies No. 54.

Bastida-Corcuera, F. D., Butler, J. E., Yahiro, S., and Corbeil, L. B. (1999). Differential complement activation by bovine IgG2 allotypes. *Vet. Immunol. Immunopathol.* 71, 115–123. doi: 10.1016/S0165-2427(99)00095-1

Bekker PM. The history of dipping. *Veld.* 1960;**20**:1–5.

Bennett, G. F. (1969). Boophilus microplus (Acarina: Ixodidae): experimental infestations on cattle restrained from grooming. *Exp. Parasitol.* 26, 323–328. doi: 10.1016/0014-4894(69)90125-8

Benson, A. K., Kelly, S. A., Legge, R., Ma, F., Low, S. J., Kim, J., et al. (2010). Individuality in gut microbiota composition is a complex polygenic trait shaped by multiple environmental and host genetic factors. *Proc. Natl. Acad. Sci. U.S.A.* 107, 18933–18938. doi: 10.1073/pnas.1007028107

Ben-Yakir, D., Fox, C. J., Homer, J. T., and Barker, R. W. (1987). Quantification of host immunoglobulin in the hemolymph of ticks. *J. Parasitol.* 73, 669–671. doi: 10.2307/3282157

Bézie, S., Picarda, E., Tesson, L., Renaudin, K., Durand, J., Ménoret, S., et al. (2015). Fibrinogen-like protein 2/fibroleukin induces long-term allograft survival in a rat model through regulatory B Cells. *PLoS ONE* 10:e0119686. doi: 10.1371/journal.pone.0119686

Biegelmeyer, P., Nizoli, L. Q., da Silva, S. S., dos Santos, T. R. B., Dionello, N. J. L., Gulias-Gomes, C. C., et al. (2015). Bovine genetic resistance effects on biological traits of *Rhipicephalus (Boophilus) microplus*. *Vet. Parasitol.* 208, 231–237. doi: 10.1016/j.vetpar.2015.01.010

Blakeslee, D., Butler, J. E., and Stone, W. H. (1971). Serum antigens of cattle. II. Immunogenetics of two immunoglobulin allotypes. *J. Immunol.* 107, 227–235.

Bock RE, de Vos AJ, Kinston TG, McLellan DJ. The effect of breed of cattle on innate resistance to infection with *Babesia bovis*, *Babesia bigemina*, and *Anaplasma marginale* . *Aust Vet J.* 1997;**5**:337–340.

Bolormaa, S., Hayes, B. J., Hawken, R. J., Zhang, Y., Reverter, A., and Goddard, M. E. (2011). Detection of chromosome segments of zebu and taurine origin and their effect on beef production and growth. *J. Anim. Sci.* 89, 2050–2060. doi: 10.2527/jas.2010-3363

Borges, L. M. F., de Oliveira Filho, J. G., Ferreira, L. L., Louly, C. C. B., Pickett, J. A., and Birkett, M. A. (2015). Identification of non-host semiochemicals for the brown dog tick, *Rhipicephalus sanguineus* sensu lato (Acari: Ixodidae), from tick-resistant beagles, Canis lupus familiaris. *Ticks Tick Borne Dis.* 6, 676–682. doi: 10.1016/j.ttbdis.2015.05.014

Bram RA. Tick-borne livestock diseases and their vectors. 1. The global problem. *Wld Anim Rev, (FAO)* 1983;**36**:1–5

Bram RA, George JE, Reichard RE, Tabachnick WJ. The threat of foreign arthropod-borne pathogens to livestock in the United States. *J Med Entomol.* 2002;**39**:405–416.

Bramble, B. J., 1989. An environmentalist view of pest management and the Green Revolution. Tropical Pest Management, vol. 35, no. 3, pp. 228-230.

Branagan D. Observations on the development and survival of the ixodid ticks *Rhipicephalus appendiculatus* (Neumann 1901) under quasi natural conditions in Kenya. *Trop Anim Health Prod.* 1973;**5**(3):153–165. doi: 10.1007/BF02251384.

Burger, T. D., Shao, R., and Barker, S. C. (2014). Phylogenetic analysis of mitochondrial genome sequences indicates that the cattle tick, *Rhipicephalus (Boophilus) microplus*, contains a cryptic species. *Mol. Phylogenet. Evol.* 76, 241–253. doi: 10.1016/j.ympev.2014.03.017

Butler, J. E., Navarro, P., and Heyermann, H. (1994). Heterogeneity of bovine IgG2. VI. Comparative specificity of monoclonal and polyclonal capture antibodies for IgG2a (A1) and IgG2a (A2). *Vet. Immunol. Immunopathol.* 40, 119–133. doi: 10.1016/0165-2427(94)90028-0

Cardoso, F. F., Gomes, C. C. G., Sollero, B. P., Oliveira, M. M., Roso, V. M., Piccoli, M. L., et al. (2015). Genomic prediction for tick resistance in Braford and Hereford cattle. *J. Anim. Sci.* 93, 2693–2705. doi: 10.2527/jas.2014-8832

Carretta, M. D., Hidalgo, A. I., Burgos, J., Opazo, L., Castro, L., Hidalgo, M. A., et al. (2016). Butyric acid stimulates bovine neutrophil functions and potentiates the effect of platelet activating factor. *Vet.*

Immunol. Immunopathol. 176, 18–27. doi: 10.1016/j.vetimm.2016.05.002

Carvalho, W. A., Bechara, G. H., More, D. D., Ferreira, B. R., da Silva, J. S., and de Miranda Santos, I. K. (2008). *Rhipicephalus (Boophilus) microplus*: distinct acute phase proteins vary during infestations according to the genetic composition of the bovine hosts, *Bos taurus* and *Bos indicus*. *Exp. Parasitol.* 118, 587–591. doi: 10.1016/j.exppara.2007.10.006

Carvalho, W. A., Domingues, R., de Azevedo Prata, M. C., da Silva, M. V. G. B., de Oliveira, G. C., Guimarães, S. E. F., et al. (2014). Microarray analysis of tick-infested skin in resistant and susceptible cattle confirms the role of inflammatory pathways in immune activation and larval rejection. *Vet. Parasitol.* 205, 307–317. doi: 10.1016/j.vetpar.2014.07.018

Carvalho, W. A., Franzin, A. M., Abatepaulo, A. R. R., de Oliveira, C. J. F., Moré, D. D., da Silva, J. S., et al. (2010a). Modulation of cutaneous inflammation induced by ticks in contrasting phenotypes of infestation in bovines. *Vet. Parasitol.* 167, 260–273. doi: 10.1016/j.vetpar.2009.09.028

Carvalho, W. A., Ianella, P., Arnoldi, F. G. C., Caetano, A. R., Maruyama, S. R., Ferreira, B. R., et al. (2011). Haplotypes of the bovine IgG2 heavy gamma chain in tick-resistant and tick-susceptible breeds of cattle. *Immunogenetics* 63, 319–324. doi: 10.1007/s00251-011-0515-y

Carvalho, W. A., Maruyama, S. R., Franzin, A. M., Abatepaulo, A. R. R., Anderson, J. M., Ferreira, B. R., et al. (2010b). *Rhipicephalus (Boophilus) microplus*: clotting time in tick-infested skin varies according to local inflammation and gene expression patterns in tick salivary glands. *Exp. Parasitol.* 124, 428–435.

Chaka G, Madder M, Seybroeck N, Tempia S, Tona K, Berkvens D. Determination of the physiological age of *Rhipicephalus appendiculatus* (Acari: Ixodidae) *Syst Appl Acarol Spec Publ.* 2001;**10**:1–16.

Chiera JW, Cunningham MP, Dolan TT, Newson RM, Radley DE, Young AS. Survival of *Rhipicephalus appendiculatus* (Acari: Ixodidae) and persistence of *Theileria parva* (Apicomplexa: Theileridae) in the field. *Int J Parasitol.* 1984;**14**:48–49.

Constantinoiu, C. C., Jackson, L. A., Jorgensen, W. K., Lew-Tabor, A. E., Piper, E. K., Mayer, D. G., et al. (2010). Local immune response against larvae of *Rhipicephalus (Boophilus) microplus* in *Bos taurus indicus* and *Bos taurus taurus* cattle. *Int. J. Parasitol.* 40, 865–875. doi: 10.1016/j.ijpara.2010.01.004

Constantinoiu, C. C., Jonsson, N. N., Jorgensen, W. K., Jackson, L. A., Piper, E. K., and Lew-Tabor, A. E. (2013). Immuno-fluorescence staining patterns of leukocyte subsets in the skin of taurine and indicine cattle. *Res. Vet. Sci.* 95, 854–860. doi: 10.1016/j.rvsc.2013.08.014

CRC-VT. *Australian Government Cooperative Research Centres Program.* 2001. Research Program: Vaccine Applications, Tick Fever.

Cruz, A. P. R., Silva, S. S., Mattos, R. T., Da Silva Vaz Jr, I., Masuda, A., and Ferreira, C. A. S. (2008). Comparative IgG recognition of tick extracts by sera of experimentally infested bovines. *Vet. Parasitol.* 158, 152–158. doi: 10.1016/j.vetpar.2008.08.016

Cui, Y., and Yu, L. (2016). Application of the CRISPR/Cas9 gene editing technique to research on functional genomes of parasites. *Parasitol. Int.* 65, 641–644. doi: 10.1016/j.parint.2016.08.011

da Silva, E. Z. M., Jamur, M. C., and Oliver, C. (2014). Mast cell function. *J. Histochem. Cytochem.* 62, 698–738. doi: 10.1369/0022155414545334

Davis, T. S., Crippen, T. L., Hofstetter, R. W., and Tomberlin, J. K. (2013). Microbial volatile emissions as insect semiochemicals. *J. Chem. Ecol.* 39, 840–859. doi: 10.1007/s10886-013-0306-z

de Castro, J. J., Cunningham, M. P., Dolan, T. T., Dransfield, R. D., Newson, R. M., and Young, A. S. (1985). Effects on cattle of artificial infestations with the tick *Rhipicephalus appendiculatus*. *Parasitology* 90, 21–33. doi: 10.1017/S0031182000048988

de Castro, J. J., and Newson, R. M. (1993). Host resistance in cattle tick control. *Parasitol. Today* 9, 13–17. doi: 10.1016/0169-4758(93)90154-8

de la Fuente, J., and Contreras, M. (2015). Tick vaccines: current status and future directions. *Expert Rev. Vaccines* 14, 1367–1376. doi: 10.1586/14760584.2015.1076339

de la Fuente, J., Kopacek, P., Lew-Tabor, A., and Maritz-Olivier, C. (2016). Strategies for new and improved vaccines against ticks and tick-borne diseases. *Parasite Immunol.* 38, 754–769. doi: 10.1111/pim.12339

de Oliveira Filho, J. G., Sarria, A. L. F., Ferreira, L. L., Caulfield, J. C., Powers, S. J., Pickett, J. A., et al. (2016). Quantification of brown dog tick repellents, 2-hexanone and benzaldehyde, and release from tick-resistant beagles, *Canis lupus* familiaris. *J. Chromatogr. B* 1022, 64–69. doi: 10.1016/j.jchromb.2016.03.014

de Oliveira, M. N. V., Jewell, K. A., Freitas, F. S., Benjamin, L. A., Tótola, M. R., Borges, A. C., et al. (2013). Characterizing the microbiota across the gastrointestinal tract of a Brazilian Nelore steer. *Vet. Microbiol.* 164, 307–314. doi: 10.1016/j.vetmic.2013.02.013

Domingues, R., Wohlres-Viana, S., Reis, D. R., Teixeira, H. C., Ferreira, A. P., Guimarães, S. E., et al. (2014). Expression of immune response genes in peripheral blood of cattle infested with Rhipicephalus microplus. *Genet. Mol. Res.* 13, 4013–4021. doi: 10.4238/2014.May.23.12

Doube, B. M., and Wharton, R. H. (1980). The effect of locality, breed and previous tick experience on seasonal changes in the resistance of cattle to *Boophilus microplus* (Ixodoidea: Ixodidae). *Experientia* 36, 1178–1179. doi: 10.1007/BF01976112

Doube BM, Kemp DH. Paralysis of cattle by *Ixodes holocyclus* Neumann. *Aust J Agric Res.* 1975;**26**(3):635–640. doi: 10.1071/AR9750635.

Dowd, S. E., Callaway, T. R., Wolcott, R. D., Sun, Y., McKeehan, T., Hagevoort, R. G., et al. (2008). Evaluation of the bacterial diversity in the feces of cattle using 16S rDNA bacterial tag-encoded FLX amplicon pyrosequencing (bTEFAP). *BMC Microbiol.* 8:125. doi: 10.1186/1471-2180-8-125

Drummond RO. Tick-borne livestock diseases and their vectors. Chemical control of ticks. *Wld Anim Rev, (FAO)* 1983;**36**:28–33.

Duncan IM. Tick control on cattle with flumethrin pour-on through a Duncan applicator. *J S Afr Vet Assoc.* 1991;**63**(3):125–127.

Durso, L. M., Harhay, G. P., Smith, T. P. L., Bono, J. L., DeSantis, T. Z., Harhay, D. M., et al. (2010). Animal-to-animal variation in fecal microbial fiversity among beef cattle. *Appl. Environ. Microbiol.* 76, 4858–4862. doi: 10.1128/AEM.00207-10

Durso, L. M., Wells, J. E., Harhay, G. P., Rice, W. C., Kuehn, L., Bono, J. L., et al. (2012). Comparison of bacterial communities in faeces of beef cattle fed diets containing corn and wet distillers' grain with solubles. *Letts Appl. Microbiol.* 55, 109–114. doi: 10.1111/j.1472-765X.2012.03265.x

Engracia Filho, J. R., Araújo, C. D., Pinto, G. N., Mendes, Y. H., and Bechara, G. H. (2017). Cellular response in the tick feeding site in crossbred cattle artificially infested by *Rhipicephalus microplus*. *Exp. Appl. Acarol.* 72, 171–178. doi: 10.1007/s1

Estrada-Peña, A., Bouattour, A., Camicas, J. L., Guglielmone, A., Horak, I., Jongejan, F., et al. (2006). The known distribution and ecological preferences of the tick subgenus Boophilus (Acari: Ixodidae) in Africa and Latin America. *Exp. Appl. Acarol.* 38, 219–235. doi: 10.1007/s10493-006-0003-5 0493-017-0143-9

Estrada-Peña A. Forecasting habitat suitability for ticks and prevention of tick-borne diseases. *Vet Parasitol.* 2001;**98**(1-3):111–132. doi: 10.1016/S0304-4017(01)00426-5.

FAO. 1998. (Available from: http://www.fao.org/ag/AGA/AGAH/PD/pages/tick01.htm

Feldman-Muhsam, B. (1964). Laboratory colonies of Rhipicephalus. *Bull. World Health Organ*. 31, 587–589.

Fernandes FF. Toxicological effects and resistance to pyrethroids in *Boophilus microplus* from Goias. *Brazil Arq Bras Med Vet Zoot.* 2001;**53**:538–543.

Ferreira, L. L., Soares, S. F., de Oliveira Filho, J. G., Oliveira, T. T., Pérez de León, A. A., and Borges, L. M. F. (2015). Role of *Rhipicephalus microplus* cheliceral receptors in gustation and host differentiation. *Ticks Tick Borne Dis*. 6, 228–233. doi: 10.1016/j.ttbdis.2014.12.008

Fischer, S., Trefz, P., Bergmann, A., Steffens, M., Ziller, M., Miekisch, W., et al. (2015). Physiological variability in volatile organic compounds (VOCs) in exhaled breath and released from faeces due to nutrition and somatic growth in a standardized caprine animal model. *J. Breath Res*. 9:027108. doi: 10.1088/1752-7155/9/2/027108

Foster, V and Mourato, S., 1997. Behavioural consistency, statistical specification and validity in the contingent ranking method: Evidence from a survey on the impacts of pesticide use in the U.K. CSERGE Working Paper GEC 97-07

Frans J. *Final Report, Integrated Control of Ticks and Tick-Born Diseases (ICTTD)* 2000. p. 4. (Available from: http://www.uu.nl/tropical.ticks)

Franzin, A. M., Maruyama, S. R., Garcia, G. R., Oliveira, R. P., Ribeiro, J. M. C., Bishop, R., et al. (2017). Immune and biochemical responses in skin differ between bovine hosts genetically susceptible and resistant to the cattle tick *Rhipicephalus microplus*. *Parasit. Vectors* 10:51. doi: 10.1186/s13071-016-1945-z

Frisch, J. E. (1999). Towards a permanent solution for controlling cattle ticks. *Int. J. Parasitol.* 29, 57–71. doi: 10.1016/S0020-7519(98)00177-5

Furman DP, Loomis EC. *Bulletin of the California Insect Survey.* Vol. 25. California: University of California Press; 1984. The Ticks of California (Acari: Ixodida) pp. 1–239. University of California Publications.

Garcia, G. R., Maruyama, S. R., Nelson, K. T., Ribeiro, J. M. C., Gardinassi, L. G., Maia, A. A. M., et al. (2017). Immune recognition of salivary proteins from the cattle tick *Rhipicephalus microplus* differs according to the genotype of the bovine host. *Parasit. Vectors* 10:144. doi: 10.1186/s13071-017-2077-9

García-García JC, Montero C, Redondo M, Vargas M, Canales M, Boue O, Rodríguez M, Joglar M, Machado H, González IL, et al. Control of ticks resistant to immunization with Bm86 in cattle vaccinated with the recombinant antigen Bm95 isolated from the cattle tick, *Boophilus microplus* . *Vaccine.* 2000;**18**(21):2275–2287. doi: 10.1016/S0264-410X(99)00548-4.

Gasparin, G., Miyata, M., Coutinho, L. L., Martinez, M. L., Teodoro, R. L., Furlong, J., et al. (2007). Mapping of quantitative trait loci controlling tick *Riphicephalus (Boophilus) microplus* resistance on bovine chromosomes 5, 7and 14G. *Anim. Genet.* 38, 453–459. doi: 10.1111/j.1365-2052.2007.01634.x

George JE. Present and future technologies for tick control. *Ann N Y Acad Sci.* 2000;**916**:583–588.

George JE, Pound JM, Davey RB. Chemical control of ticks on cattle and the resistance of these parasites to acaricides. *Parasitology.* 2004;**129**(7):S353–S366. doi: 10.1017/S0031182003004682.

Gladney WJ, Grabbe RR, Ernst SE, Oehler DD. The gulf coast tick: evidence of a pheromone produced by males. *J Med Ent.* 1974;**11**:303–306.

Gong, H., Qin, S., Wan, X., Zhang, H., Zhou, Y., Cao, J., et al. (2014). Immunoglobulin G binding protein (IGBP) from *Rhipicephalus haemaphysaloides*: identification, expression, and binding specificity. *Parasitol. Res.* 113, 4387–4395. doi: 10.1007/s00436-014-4115-2

Graf JF, Gogolewski R, Leach-Bing N, Sabatini GA, Molento MB, Bordin EL, Arantes GJ. Tick control: an industry point of view. *Parasitology.* 2004;**129**(Suppl.):S427–S442. doi: 10.1017/S0031182004006079.

Graham, H. T., Lowry, O. H., Wheelwright, F., Lenz, M. A., and Parish, H. H. (1955). Distribution of histamine among leukocytes and platelets. *Blood* 10:467.

Graham OH, Hourrigan JL. Eradication programs for the arthropod parasites of livestock. *J Med Ent.* 1977;**13**:629–658.

Gregson, J. D. (1941). Host immunity to ticks (Acarina). *J. Entomol. Soc.* 38, 12–13.

Grisi L, Massard CL, Moya BGE, Pereira JB. Impacto econômico das principais ectoparasitoses em bovinos no Brasil. *A Hora Veterinária.* 2002;**21**:8–10.

Gudderra, N. P., Sonenshine, D. E., Apperson, C. S., and Roe, R. M. (2002). Hemolymph proteins in ticks. *J. Insect Physiol.* 48, 269–278. doi: 10.1016/S0022-1910(02)00050-1

Hayman RH. The development of the Australian milking zebu. *Wld Anim Rev, (FAO)* 1974;**11**:31–35.

Hewetson, R. W. (1972). "The inheritance of resistance by cattle to cattle tick," in *Australian Veterinary Association Conference Paper* (Brisbane, QLD).

Heyermann, H., and Butler, J. E. (1987). the heterogeneity of bovine IgG2—IV. Structural differences between IgG2a molecules of the A1 and A2 allotypes. *Mol. Immunol.* 24, 1327–1334. doi: 10.1016/0161-5890(87)90128-3

Hogarth, P. M. (2002). Fc receptors are major mediators of antibody based inflammation in autoimmunity. *Curr. Opin. Immunol.* 14, 798–802. doi: 10.1016/S0952-7915(02)00409-0

Jenkins MC. Advances and prospects for subunit vaccines against protozoa of veterinary importance. *Vet Parasitol.* 2001;**101**(3-4):291–310. doi: 10.1016/S0304-4017(01)00557-X.

Jones, K. E., Patel, N. G., Levy, M. A., Storeygard, A., Balk, D., Gittleman, J. L., et al. (2008). Global trends in emerging infectious diseases. *Nature* 451, 990–993. doi: 10.1038/nature06536

Jonsson, N. N., Piper, E. K., and Constantinoiu, C. C. (2014). Host resistance in cattle to infestation with the cattle tick *Rhipicephalus microplus*. *Parasite Immunol.* 36, 553–559. doi: 10.1111/pim.12140

Kaaya GP, Hassan S. Entomogenous fungi as promising biopesticides for tick control. *Exp Appl Acarol.* 2000;**24**(12):913–926. doi: 10.1023/A:1010722914299.

Kacskovics, I., and Butler, J. E. (1996). The heterogeneity of bovine IgG2—VIII. The complete cDNA sequence of bovine IgG2a (A2) and an IgG1. *Mol. Immunol.* 33, 189–195. doi: 10.1016/0161-5890(95)00107-7

Karasuyama, H., Wada, T., Yoshikawa, S., and Obata, K. (2011). Emerging roles of basophils in protective immunity against parasites. *Trends Immunol.* 32, 125–130. doi: 10.1016/j.it.2010.11.006

Kashino, S. S., Resende, J., Sacco, A. M. S., Rocha, C., Proenca, L., Carvalho, W. A., et al. (2005). *Boophilus microplus*: the pattern of bovine immunoglobulin isotype responses to high and low tick infestations. *Exp. Parasitol.* 110, 12–21. doi: 10.1016/j.exppara.2005.01.006

Kaufman, W. R. (1989). Tick-host interaction: a synthesis of current concepts. *Parasitol. Today* 5, 47–56. doi: 10.1016/0169-4758(89)90191-9

Kemp, D. H., and Bourne, A. (1980). *Boophilus microplus*: the effect of histamine on the attachment of cattle-tick larvae–studies *in vivo* and *in vitro*. *Parasitology* 80, 487–496. doi: 10.1017/S0031182000000950

Kemp, D. H., Koudstaal, D., Roberts, J. A., and Kerr, J. D. (1976). Boophilus microplus: the effect of host resistance on larval attachments and growth. *Parasitology* 73, 123–136. doi: 10.1017/S0031182000051386

Kishore, U., Gaboriaud, C., Waters, P., Shrive, A. K., Greenhough, T. J., Reid, K. B. M., et al. (2004). C1q and tumor necrosis factor superfamily: modularity and versatility. *Trends Immunol.* 25, 551–561. doi: 10.1016/j.it.2004.08.006

Klompen JSH, Black WCIV, Keirans JE, Oliver JHJr. Evolution of ticks. *Annu Rev Entomol.* 1996;**41**(1):141–161. doi: 10.1146/annurev.en.41.010196.001041.

Knight, K. L., Suter, M., and Becker, R. S. (1988). Genetic engineering of bovine Ig. Construction and characterization of hapten-binding bovine/murine chimeric IgE, IgA, IgG1, IgG2, and IgG3 molecules. *J. Immunol.* 140, 3654–3659.

Kongsuwan, K., Josh, P., Colgrave, M. L., Bagnall, N. H., Gough, J., Burns, B., et al. (2010). Activation of several key components of the epidermal differentiation pathway in cattle following infestation with the cattle tick, *Rhipicephalus (Boophilus) microplus*. *Int. J. Parasitol.* 40, 499–507. doi: 10.1016/j.ijpara.2009.10.013

L'Hostis M, Seegers H. Tick-borne parasitic diseases in cattle: current knowledge and prospective risk analysis related to the ongoing evolution in French cattle farming systems. *Vet Res.* 2002;**33**(5):599–611. doi: 10.1051/vetres:2002041.

Laffont CM, Alvinerie M, Bousquet-Melou A, Toutain PL. Licking behavior and environmental contamination arising from pour-on ivermectin for cattle. *Int J Parasitol.* 2001;**31**(14):1687–1692. doi: 10.1016/S0020-7519(01)00285-5.

Latif AA, Pegram RG. Naturally acquired host-resistance in tick control in Africa. *Insect Sci & Appl.* 1992;**13**:505–513.

Lew-Tabor, A. E., and Rodriguez Valle, M. (2016). A review of reverse vaccinology approaches for the development of vaccines against ticks and tick borne diseases. *Ticks Tick Borne Dis.* 7, 573–585. doi: 10.1016/j.ttbdis.2015.12.012

Lodos J, Boue O, de la Fuente JA. Model to simulate the effect of vaccination against Boophilus ticks on cattle. *Vet Parasitol.* 2000;**87**(4):315–326. doi: 10.1016/S0304-4017(99)00187-9.

Louly, C. C. B., Soares, S. F., da Nóbrega Silveira, D., Guimarães, M. S., and Borges, L. M. F. (2010). Differences in the behavior of Rhipicephalus sanguineus tested against resistant and susceptible dogs. *Exp. Appl. Acarol.* 51, 353–362. doi: 10.1007/s10493-009-9334-3

Low, V. L., Tay, S. T., Kho, K. L., Koh, F. X., Tan, T. K., Lim, Y. A. L., et al. (2015). Molecular characterisation of the tick *Rhipicephalus microplus* in Malaysia: new insights into the cryptic diversity and distinct genetic assemblages throughout the world. *Parasit. Vectors* 8:341. doi: 10.1186/s13071-015-0956-5

Lundholm, E., 1987. Thinning of eggshells in birds by DDT: Mode of action on the eggshell gland. Comparative Biochemistry and Physiology, vol. 88, pp. 1-22.

Lysyk TJ, Majak W, Veira DM. Prefeeding *Dermacentor andersoni* (Acari: Ixodidae) on cattle with prior tick exposure may inhibit detection of tick paralysis by using hamster bioassay. *J Med Entomol.* 2005;**42**(3):376–382.

Machado, M. A., Azevedo, A. L., Teodoro, R. L., Pires, M. A., Peixoto, M. G., de Freitas, C., et al. (2010). Genome wide scan for quantitative trait loci affecting tick resistance in cattle (*Bos taurus* x *Bos indicus*). *BMC Genomics* 11:280. doi: 10.1186/1471-2164-11-280

Mans, B. J., Anderson, J. F., Francischetti, I. M. B., Valenzuela, J. G., Schwan, T. G., Pham, V. M., et al. (2008). Comparative sialomics between hard and soft ticks: implications for the evolution of blood-feeding behavior. *Insect Biochem. Mol. Biol.* 38, 42–58. doi: 10.1016/j.ibmb.2007.09.003

Mao, S., Zhang, M., Liu, J., and Zhu, W. (2015). Characterising the bacterial microbiota across the gastrointestinal tracts of dairy cattle: membership and potential function. *Sci. Rep.* 5:16116. doi: 10.1038/srep16116

Mapholi, N. O., Maiwashe, A., Matika, O., Riggio, V., Bishop, S. C., MacNeil, M. D., et al. (2016). Genome-wide association study of tick resistance in South African *Nguni cattle*. *Ticks Tick Borne Dis.* 7, 487–497. doi: 10.1016/j.ttbdis.2016.02.005

Mapholi, N. O., Marufu, M. C., Maiwashe, A., Banga, C. B., Muchenje, V., MacNeil, M. D., et al. (2014). Towards a genomics approach to tick (Acari:Ixodidae) control in cattle: a review. *Ticks Tick Borne Dis*. 5, 475–483. doi: 10.1016/j.ttbdis.2014.04.006

Marchant, J. H., Hudson, R., Carter, S. P. and Whittington, P. A., 1990. Population trends in British breeding birds. British Trust for Ornithology, Tring, Hertfordshire, U.K.

Martinez, M. L., Machado, M. A., Nascimento, C. S., Silva, M. V. G. B., Teodoro, R. L., Furlong, J., et al. (2006). Association of BoLA-DRB3.2 alleles with tick (*Boophilus microplus*) resistance in cattle. *Genet. Mol. Res.* 5, 513–524. Available online at: http://www.funpecrp.com.br/gmr/year2006/vol3-5/pdf/gmr0211.pdf

Martins JR, Corrêa BL, Cereser VH, et al. A Situation Report on Resistance to Acaricides by the Cattle Tick *Boophilus microplus* in the State of Rio Grande do Sul, Southern Brazil. In: Rodriguez CS, Fragoso SH, editors. *Resistencia y Control en Garrapatas y Moscas de Importancia Veterinaria III.* Acapulco, Mexico: Seminario Internacional de Parasitologia Animal; 1995. pp. 1–8.

Marufu, M. C., Chimonyo, M., Mans, B. J., and Dzama, K. (2013). Cutaneous hypersensitivity responses to *Rhipicephalus tick* larval antigens in pre-sensitized cattle. *Ticks Tick Borne Dis.* 4, 311–316. doi: 10.1016/j.ttbdis.2012.12.001

Marufu, M. C., Dzama, K., and Chimonyo, M. (2014). Cellular responses to *Rhipicephalus microplus* infestations in pre-sensitised cattle with differing phenotypes of infestation. *Exp. Appl. Acarol.* 62, 241–252. doi: 10.1007/s10493-013-9723-5

Marufu, M. C., Qokweni, L., Chimonyo, M., and Dzama, K. (2011). Relationships between tick counts and coat characteristics in Nguni and *Bonsmara cattle* reared on semiarid rangelands in South

Africa. *Ticks Tick Borne Dis.* 2, 172–177. doi: 10.1016/j.ttbdis.2011.07.001

Mason IL. Maintaining crossbred populations of dairy cattle in the tropics. *Wld Anim Rev, (FAO)* 1974;**11**:36–43.

Mason, C. F., Ford, T. C., and Last, N. 1., 1986. Organochlorine residues in British Otters. Bulletin of Environmental Contamination and Toxicology, vol. 36, pp. 429- 36.

Matsuda, H., Nakano, T., Kiso, Y., and Kitamura, Y. (1987). Normalization of anti-tick response of mast cell-deficient W/Wv mice by intracutaneous injection of cultured mast cells. *J. Parasitol.* 73, 155–160. doi: 10.2307/3282361

Matthewson MD, Baker JAF. Arsenic resistance in species of multihost ticks in the Republic of South Africa and Swaziland. *J S Afr Vet Assoc.* 1975;**46**:341–344.

Mbati PA, Hlatshwayo M, Mtshali MS, Mogaswane KR, de Waal TD, Dipeolu OO. Ticks and tick-borne diseases of livestock belonging to resource-poor farmers in the eastern Free State of South Africa. *Exp Appl Acarol.* 2002;**28**(1-4):217–224. doi: 10.1023/A:1025306701803.

Millar JA, Davey RB, Oehler DD, Pound JM, George JE. The Ivermectin was delivered orally in the case of *Boophilus annulatus* on cattle in South Texas. *J Econ Entomol.* 2001;**94**:1622–1627.

Mohler JR. *The Cattle Tick in Its Relation to Southern Agriculture.* Washington D.C: 1906. p. 258. United States Department, Agriculture Farmer's Bulletin.

Moraes, F. R., Moraes, J. R. E., Costa, A. J., Rocha, U. F., and Ardisson, F. A. (1992). A Comparative study of lesions eauscd by different parasitic stages of *Boophilus microplus* (Canestrini) in the skins of naturally inffcstcd taurine and zebuine hosts. The correlation of tick resistance with mast cell counts in the host's skin. *Braz. J. Vet Res. Anim.* 29, 378–383 Suplemento.

Morel PC. Reflexions on epizootiology of the European bovine babesiosis with *Babesia divergens* . *Bull Acad Vét Fr.* 1980;**53**:451–456.

Murray, A., 1985. Acute and residual toxicity of a new pyrethroid insecticide, WL 85871, to honey bees. Bulletin of Environmental Contamination and Toxicology, vol. 34, pp. 560-64.

Mwase ET, Pegram RG, Mathers TN. New Strategies for Controlling Ticks. In: Curtis CF, editor. *Appropriate Technology in Vector Control.* FL, USA: Boca Raton; 1990. pp. 93–102.

Nascimento, C. S., Machado, M. A., Guimarães, S. E., Guimarães, M. F., Peixoto, J. O., Furlong, J., et al. (2010). Differential expression of genes in resistant versus susceptible Gyr x Holstein cattle challenged with the tick *Rhipicephalus (Boophilus) microplus*. *Genet. Mol. Res.* 9, 1974–1979. doi: 10.4238/vol9-4gmr905

Nascimento, C. S., Machado, M. A., Guimarães, S. E., Martins, M. F., Peixoto, J. O., Furlong, J., et al. (2011). Expressed sequenced tags profiling of resistant and susceptible Gyr x Holstein cattle infested with the tick *Rhipicephalus (Boophilus) microplus*. *Genet. Mol. Res.* 10, 3803–3816. doi: 10.4238/2011.November.8.3

Nolan J. Acaricide resistence in single and multi-host ticks and strategies for control. *Parasitol.* 1990;**32**:145–153.

Norval RAI, Lawrence JA, Young AS, Perry BD, Dolan TT, Scott J. *Theileria parva*: influence of vector, parasite and host relationships on the nature and distribution of theileriosis in southern Africa. *Parasitology*. 1991;**102**:247–356.

Nuttall, G. H. F. (1911). On the adaptation of ticks to the habits of their hosts. *Parasitology* 4, 46–67. doi: 10.1017/S0031182000002456

Ogden, N. H., and Lindsay, L. R. (2016). Effects of climate and climate change on vectors and vector-borne diseases: ticks are different. *Trends Parasitol.* 32, 646–656. doi: 10.1016/j.pt.2016.04.015

Oliver JHJr. Biology and systematics of ticks (Acari: Ixidida) *Annu Rev Ecol Syst.* 1989;**20**(1):397–430. doi: 10.1146/annurev.es.20.110189.002145.

Opdebeeck, J. P., and Daly, K. E. (1990). Immune responses of infested and vaccinated Hereford cattle to antigens of the cattle tick, *Boophilus microplus*. *Vet. Immunol. Immunopathol.* 25, 99–108. doi: 10.1016/0165-2427(90)90113-7

Osterkamp, J., Wahl, U., Schmalfuss, G., and Haas, W. (1999). Host-odour recognition in two tick species is coded in a blend of vertebrate volatiles. *J. Comp. Physiol. A* 185, 59–67. doi: 10.1007/s003590050366

Paesen, G. C., Adams, P. L., Harlos, K., Nuttall, P. A., and Stuart, D. I. (1999). Tick histamine-binding proteins: isolation, cloning, and three-dimensional structure. *Mol. Cell* 3, 661–671. doi: 10.1016/S1097-2765(00)80359-7

Perry BD, Musisi FL, Pegram RG, Schels HF. Assessment of enzootic stability to tick-borne diseases in Zambia. *Wld Anim Rev, (FAO)* 1985;**56**:24–32.

Pingali, P. L and Rosegrant, M. W. 1994. Confronting the environmental consequences of the green revolution in Asia. EPTD Discussion Paper, No.2, International Food Policy Research Institute, Washington.

Piper, E. K., Jackson, L. A., Bagnall, N., Kongsuwan, K., Lew, A. E., and Jonsson, N. N. (2008). Gene expression in skin of *Bos taurus* and *Bos indicus* cattle infested with the cattle tick. *Vet. Immunol. Immunopathol.* 126, 110–119. doi: 10.1016/j.vetimm.2008.06.011

Piper, E. K., Jackson, L. A., Bielefeldt-Ohmann, H., Gondro, C., Lew-Tabor, A. E., and Jonsson, N. N. (2010). Tick-susceptible *Bos taurus* cattle display an increased cellular response at the site of larval *Rhipicephalus (Boophilus) microplus* attachment, compared with tick-resistant *Bos indicus* cattle. *Int. J. Parasitol.* 40, 865–875. doi: 10.1016/j.ijpara.2009.09.009

Piper, E. K., Jonsson, N. N., Gondro, C., Lew-Tabor, A. E., Moolhuijzen, P., Vance, M. E., et al. (2009). Immunological profiles of *Bos taurus* and *Bos indicus* cattle infested with the cattle tick, *Rhipicephalus (Boophilus) microplus*. *Clin. Vaccine Immunol.* 16, 1074–1086. doi: 10.1128/CVI.00157-09

Piper, E. K., Jonsson, N. N., Gondro, C., Vance, M. E., Lew-Tabor, A., and Jackson, L. A. (2017). Peripheral cellular and humoral responses to infestation with the cattle tick *Rhipicephalus microplus* in Santa Gertrudis cattle. *Parasite Immunol.* 39:e12402. doi: 10.1111/pim.12402

Porto Neto, L. R., Bunch, R. J., Harrison, B. E., and Barendse, W. (2011a). DNA variation in the gene ELTD1 is associated with tick burden in cattle. *Anim. Genet.* 42, 50–55. doi: 10.1111/j.1365-2052.2010.02120.x

Porto Neto, L. R., Bunch, R. J., Harrison, B. E., Prayaga, K. C., and Barendse, W. (2010a). Haplotypes that include the integrin alpha 11 gene are associated with tick burden in cattle. *BMC Genet.* 11:55. doi: 10.1186/1471-2156-11-55

Porto Neto, L. R., Jonsson, N. N., D'Occhio, M. J., and Barendse, W. (2011b). Molecular genetic approaches for identifying the basis of variation in resistance to tick infestation in cattle. *Vet. Parasitol.* 180, 165–172. doi: 10.1016/j.vetpar.2011.05.048

Porto Neto, L. R., Jonsson, N. N., Ingham, A., Bunch, R. J., Harrison, B. E., and Barendse, W. (2012). The RIPK2 gene: a positional candidate for tick burden supported by genetic associations in cattle and immunological response of knockout mouse. *Immunogenetics* 64, 379–388. doi: 10.1007/s00251-012-0601-9

Porto Neto, L. R., Piper, E. K., Jonsson, N. N., Barendse, W., and Gondro, C. (2010b). "Meta-analysis of genome wide association and gene expression studies to identify candidate genes for tick burden in cattle," in *9th World Congress of Genetics Applied to Livestock Production* (Leipzig), 0664.

Prayaga, K. C., Corbet, N. J., Johnston, D. J., Wolcott, M. L., Fordyce, G., and Burrow, H. M. (2009). Genetics of adaptive traits in heifers and their relationship to growth, pubertal and carcass traits in two tropical beef cattle genotypes. *Anim. Prod. Sci.* 49, 413–425. doi: 10.1071/EA08247

Prokop-Prigge, K. A., Mansfield, C. J., Parker, M. R., Thaler, E., Grice, E. A., Wysocki, C. J., et al. (2015). Ethnic/racial and genetic influences on cerumen odorant profiles. *J. Chem. Ecol.* 41, 67–74. doi: 10.1007/s10886-014-0533-y

Rabbani, H., Brown, W. R., Butler, J. E., and Hammarström, L. (1997). Genetic polymorphism of the IGHG3 gene in cattle. *Immunogenetics* 46, 326–331. doi: 10.1007/s002510050279

Rechav, Y. (1987). Resistance of Brahman and Hereford Cattle to African ticks with reference to serum gamma globulin levels and blood composition. *Exp. Appl. Acarol.* 3, 219–232. doi: 10.1007/BF01270458

Regassa A. The use of herbal preparations for tick control in Western Ethiopia. *J S Afr Vet Assoc.* 2000;**71**(4):240–243.

Regitano, L. C. A., Ibelli, A. M. G., Gasparin, G., Miyata, M., Azevedo, A. L. S., Coutinho, L. L., et al. (2008). On the search for markers of tick resistance in bovines. *Dev. Biol.* 132, 225–230. Available online at: https://ainfo.cnptia.embrapa.br/digital/bitstream/item/40968/1/PROCILCAR2008.00167.pdf

Riek, R. F. (1956). Factors influencing the susceptibility of cattle to tick infestation. *Aust. Vet. J.* 32, 204–209. doi: 10.1111/j.1751-0813.1956.tb05660.x

RJ, van den Bossche P, Penzhorn BL, Sharp B. Tick, fly, and mosquito control—Lessons from the past, solutions for the future. *Vet Parasitol.* 2005;**132**(3-4):205–215. doi: 10.1016/j.vetpar.2005.07.004.

Roberts, J. A., and Kerr, J. D. (1976). *Boophilus microplus*: passive transfer of resistance in cattle. *J. Parasitol.* 62, 485–488. doi: 10.2307/3279162

Rodriguez-Valle, M., Lew-Tabor, A., Gondro, C., Moolhuijzen, P., Vance, M., Guerrero, F. D., et al. (2010). Comparative microarray analysis of *Rhipicephalus (Boophilus) microplus* expression profiles of larvae pre-attachment and feeding adult female stages on Bos indicus and Bos taurus cattle. *BMC Genomics* 11:437. doi: 10.1186/1471-2164-11-437

Rodriguez-Valle, M., Moolhuijzen, P., Piper, E. K., Weiss, O., Vance, M., Bellgard, M., et al. (2013). *Rhipicephalus microplus* lipocalins (LRMs): genomic identification and analysis of the bovine immune response using *in silico* predicted B and T cell epitopes. *Int. J. Parasitol.* 43, 739–752. doi: 10.1016/j.ijpara.2013.04.005

Rodriguez-Valle, M., Vance, M., Moolhuijzen, P. M., Tao, X., and Lew-Tabor, A. E. (2012). Differential recognition by tick-resistant cattle of the recombinantly expressed *Rhipicephalus microplus* serine protease inhibitor-3 (RMS-3). *Ticks Tick Borne Dis.* 3, 159–169. doi: 10.1016/j.ttbdis.2012.03.002

Saini, S. S., Farrugia, W., Muthusamy, N., Ramsland, P. A., and Kaushik, A. K. (2007). Structural evidence for a new IgG1 antibody sequence allele of cattle. *Scand. J. Immunol.* 65, 32–38. doi: 10.1111/j.1365-3083.2006.01865.x

Santos, I. K. F. M., Valenzuela, J. G., Ribeiro, J. M. C., Castro, M., Costa, J. N., Costa, A. M., et al. (2004). Gene discovery in Boophilus microplus, the cattle tick: the transcriptomes of ovaries, salivary glands, and hemocytes. *Ann. N. Y. Acad. Sci.* 1026, 242–246. doi: 10.1196/annals.1307.037

Schetters, T., Bishop, R., Crampton, M., Kopacek, P., Lew-Tabor, A., Maritz-Olivier, C., et al. (2016). Cattle tick vaccine researchers join forces in CATVAC. *Parasit. Vectors* 9:105. doi: 10.1186/s13071-016-1386-8

Schleger, A. V., Lincoln, D. T., and Kemp, D. H. (1981). A putative role for eosinophils in tick rejection. *Experientia* 37, 49–50. doi: 10.1007/BF01965562

Schleger, A. V., Lincoln, D. T., McKenna, R. V., Kemp, D. H., and Roberts, J. A. (1976). *Boophilus microplus*: cellular responses to larval attachment and their relationship to host resistance. *Aust. J. Biol. Sci*. 29, 499–512. doi: 10.1071/BI9760499

Shapiro, S. Z., Voigt, W. P., and Fujisaki, K. (1986). Tick antigens recognized by serum from a guinea pig resistant to infestation with the tick *Rhipicephalus appendiculatus*. *J. Parasitol*. 72, 454–463. doi: 10.2307/3281686

Shanahan GJ, Hart RJ. Change in response of *Lucilia cuprina* (Weid.) to organophosphorus insecticides in Australia. *Nature*. 1966;**212**(5069):1466–1467. doi: 10.1038/2121466b0.

Smallegange, R. C., Verhulst, N. O., and Takken, W. (2011). Sweaty skin: an invitation to bite? *Trends Parasitol*. 27, 143–148. doi: 10.1016/j.pt.2010.12.009

Snelson JT. Animal ectoparasites and disease vector causing major reduction in world food supplies. *FAO Plant Protection Bulleton*. 1975;**13**:103–114.

Snowball, G. (1956). The effect of self-licking by cattle on infestations of cattle tick, *Boophilus microplus* (Canestrini). *Aust. J. Agric. Res*. 7, 227–232. doi: 10.1071/AR9560227

Sollero, B. P., Junqueira, V. S., Gomes, C. C. G., Caetano, A. R., and Cardoso, F. F. (2017). Tag SNP selection for prediction of tick resistance in Braford and Hereford cattle breeds using Bayesian methods. *Genet. Sel. Evol.* 49:49. doi: 10.1186/s12711-017-0325-2

Solomon KR. Acaricide resistance in ticks. *Advances in Veterinary Sciences and Comparative Medicine.* 1983;**27**:273–296.

Sonenshine DE. *Biology of Ticks.* Vol. 1. New York: Oxford University Press; 1991. pp. 1–449.

Spickett AM. Acaricides and resistance. *Veterinary Ectoparasitology and Protozoology.* 1998;**1**:1–13.

Spickett AM, Fivaz BH. A survey of cattle tick control practice in the Eastern Cape Province of South Africa. *Onderstepoort J Vet Res.* 1992;**59**:203–210.

Spickett, A. M., De Klerk, D., Enslin, C. B., and Scholtz, M. M. (1989). Resistance of Nguni, Bonsmara and Hereford cattle to ticks in a Bushveld region of South Africa. *Onderstepoort J. Vet. Res.* 56, 245–250.

Springell PH. The Cattle tick in relation to animal production in Australia. *Wld Anim Rev, (FAO)* 1983;**36**:1–5.

Sseruga JN, Jonsson NN, Bock RE, More SJ. Serological evidence of exposure to tick fever organisms in young cattle on Queensland dairy farms. *Aus Vet J.* 2003;**81**:147–152.

Stewart NP, de Vos AJ. Ticks and the diseases they carry. *Queensland Agriculture Journal.* 1984;**110**:295–299.

Stewart NP, Dalgliesh RJ, Tratt T. Life-cycle of tick and tick fever parasites. *Queensland Agriculture Journal.* 1981;**107**:305–308.

Stear, M. J., Hetzel, D. J., Brown, S. C., Gershwin, L. J., Mackinnon, M. J., and Nicholas, F. W. (1990). The relationships among ecto- and endoparasite levels, class I antigens of the bovine major histocompatibility system, immunoglobulin E levels and weight gain. *Vet. Parasitol.* 34, 303–321. doi: 10.1016/0304-4017(90)90077-O

Stear, M. J., Newman, M. J., Nicholas, F. W., Brown, S. C., and Holroyd, R. G. (1984). Tick resistance and the major histocompatibility system. *Aust. J. Exp. Biol. Med. Sci.* 62, 47–52. doi: 10.1038/icb.1984.4

Stear, M. J., Nicholas, F. W., Brown, S. C., and Holroyd, R. G. (1989). Class I antigens of the bovine major histocompatibility system and resistance to the cattle tick (*Boophilus microplus*) assessed in three different seasons. *Vet. Parasitol.* 31, 303–315. doi: 10.1016/0304-4017(89)90080-0

Steiner, M., Huber, S., Harrer, A., and Himly, M. (2016). The evolution of human basophil biology from neglect towards understanding of their immune functions. *BioMed Res. Int.* 2016:16. doi: 10.1155/2016/8232830

Steullet, P., and Gnerin, P. M. (1994). Identification of vertebrate volatiles stimulating olfactory receptors on tarsus I of the tick *Amblyomma variegatum* Fabricius (Ixodidae). *J. Comp. Physiol. A* 174, 39–47. doi: 10.1007/BF00192004

Sutherst RW. Management of Arthropod Parasitism in Livestock. In: Dunsmore JP, editor. *Tropical Parasites and Parasitic Zoonosis.* Perth: Murdon University; 1983. pp. 41–56.

Sutherst RW, Jones R.J. Schnitzerling HJ. Tropical legumes of the genus *Stylosanthes* immobilize and kill cattle ticks. *Nature.* 1982;**295**:320–321. doi: 10.1038/295320a0.

Symons, D. B. A., Clarkson, C. A., and Beale, D. (1989). Structure of bovine immunoglobulin constant region heavy chain gamma 1 and gamma 2 genes. *Mol. Immunol.* 26, 841–850. doi: 10.1016/0161-5890(89)90140-5

Tatchell RJ. Ecology in relation to integrated tick management. *Insect Sci & Appl.* 1992;**13**:511–561.

Tatchell, R. J., and Bennett, G. F. (1969). *Boophilus microplus*: antihistaminic and tranquilizing drugs and cattle resistance. *Exp. Parasitol.* 26, 369–377. doi: 10.1016/0014-4894(69)90130-1

Tatchell, R. J., and Moorhouse, D. E. (1968). The feeding processes of the cattle tick *Boophilus microplus* (Canestrini). *Parasitology* 58, 441–459. doi: 10.1017/S0031182000069468

Tatchell, R. J., and Moorhouse, D. E. (1970). Neutrophils: their role in the formation of a tick feeding lesion. *Science* 167, 1002–1003. doi: 10.1126/science.167.3920.1002

Tellam RL, Kemp D, Riding G, Briscoe S, Smith D, Sharp D, Irving D, Willadsen P. Reduced oviposition of *Boophilus microplus* feeding on sheep vaccinated with vitellin. *Vet Parasitol.* 2002;**103**(1-2):141–156. doi: 10.1016/S0304-4017(01)00573-8.

Tellam, R. L., Smith, D., Kemp, D. H., and Willadsen, P. (1992). "Vaccination against ticks," in *Animal Parasite Control Utilizing Biotechnology*, ed W.K. Yong (Boca Raton, FL: CRC Press Inc.), 303–331.

Thoetkiattikul, H., Mhuantong, W., Laothanachareon, T., Tangphatsornruang, S., Pattarajinda, V., Eurwilaichitr, L., et al. (2013). Comparative analysis of microbial profiles in cow rumen fed with different dietary fiber by tagged 16S rRNA gene pyrosequencing. *Curr. Microbiol.* 67, 130–137. doi: 10.1007/s00284-013-0336-3

Trager, W. (1939). Acquired immunity to ticks. *J. Parasitol.* 25, 57–81. doi: 10.2307/3272160

Turner, L. B., Harrison, B. E., Bunch, R. J., Neto, L. R. P., Li, Y., and Barendse, W. (2010). A genome-wide association study of tick burden and milk composition in cattle. *Anim. Prod. Sci.* 50, 235–245. doi: 10.1071/AN09135

Turner HG. The tropical adaptation of beef cattle: an Australian study. *Wld Anim Rev, (FAO)* 1975;**13**:16–21.

Untalan, P. M., Pruett, J. H., and Steelman, C. D. (2007). Association of the bovine leukocyte antigen major histocompatibility complex class II DRB3*4401 allele with host resistance to the Lone Star tick, *Amblyomma americanum*. *Vet. Parasitol.* 145, 190–195. doi: 10.1016/j.vetpar.2006.12.003

Urfi, A. J., 1994. Cranes like it wet. New Scientist, 2nd July, pp. 34-35

U.S. Department of Agriculture. *Agriculture Handbook, No. 321.* Washington, D.C: 1967. Safe Use of Agricultural and Household Pesticides; p. 65.

Utech, K., Wharton, R., and Kerr, J. (1978). Resistance to *Boophilus microplus* (Canestrini) in different breeds of cattle. *Aust. J. Agric. Res.* 29, 885–895. doi: 10.1071/AR9780885

Veríssimo, C. J., Bechara, G. H., Mukai, L. S., Otsuk, I. P., and Pozzi Arcaro, J. R. (2008). Mast cell counts correlate with *Rhipicephalus (Boophilus) microplus* tick load in different cattle breeds. *Braz. J. Vet. Pathol.* 1, 81–87. Available online at: http://revistas.bvs-vet.org.br/bjvp/article/view/35972

Veríssimo, C. J., D'Agostino, S. M., Pessoa, F. F., de Toledo, L. M., and de Miranda Santos, I. K. F. (2015). Length and density of filiform tongue papillae: differences between tick-susceptible and resistant cattle may affect tick loads. *Parasit. Vectors* 8:594. doi: 10.1186/s13071-015-1196-4

Veríssimo, C. J., Nicolau, C. V. J., Cardoso, V. L., and Pinheiro, M. G. (2002). Haircoat characteristics and tick infestation on Gyr (Zebu) and crossbred (Holstein × Gyr) cattle. *Arch. Zootech.* 51, 389–392. Available online at: http://citeseerx.ist.psu.edu/viewdoc/download?doi=10.1.1.514.7304&rep=rep1&type=pdf

Wagland, B. (1978). Host resistance to cattle tick (*Boophilus microplus*) in Brahman (*Bos indicus*) cattle. III.* Growth on previously unexposed animals. *Aust. J. Agric. Res.* 29, 401–409. doi: 10.1071/AR9780401

Wambura, P. N., Gwakisa, P. S., Silayo, R. S., and Rugaimukamu, E. A. (1998). Breed-associated resistance to tick infestation in *Bos indicus* and their crosses with *Bos taurus*. *Vet. Parasitol.* 77, 63–70. doi: 10.1016/S0304-4017(97)00229-X

Wang, H., and Nuttall, P. A. (1999). Immunoglobulin-binding proteins in ticks: new target for vaccine development against a blood-feeding parasite. *Cell. Mol. Life Sci.* 56, 286–295. doi: 10.1007/s000180050430

Wang, M., Guerrero, F. D., Pertea, G., and Nene, V. M. (2007). Global comparative analysis of ESTs from the southern cattle tick, *Rhipicephalus (Boophilus) microplus*. *BMC Genomics* 8, 368–382. doi: 10.1186/1471-2164-8-368

Wang, Y. H., Reverter, A., Kemp, D., McWilliam, S. M., Ingham, A., Davis, C. A., et al. (2007). Gene expression profiling of Hereford Shorthorn cattle following challenge with *Boophilus microplus* tick larvae. *Aust. J. Exp. Agric.* 47, 1397–1407. doi: 10.1071/EA07012

Wen, T., and Rothenberg, M. E. (2016). The regulatory function of eosinophils. *Microbiol. Spectrum* 4, 1–12. doi: 10.1128/microbiolspec.MCHD-0020-2015

Wharton RH. Acaricide resistance and cattle tick control. *Aust Vet J.* 1967;**43**(9):394–398.

Wharton RH. Tick-borne livestock diseases and their vectors. Acaricide resistance and alternative methods of tick control. *Wld Anim Rev, (FAO)* 1983;**36**:34–41.

Wharton RH, Roulston WJ. Resistance of ticks to chemicals. *Annu Rev Entomol.* 1970;**15**(1):381–405. doi: 10.1146/annurev.en.15.010170.002121.

Whelen, A. C., Richardson, L. K., and Wikel, S. K. (1986). Dot-ELISA assessment of guinea pig antibody responses to repeated *Dermacentor andersoni* infestations. *J. Parasitol.* 72, 155–162. doi: 10.2307/3281809

Wikel, S. K. (1982). Immune resonses to arthropods and their products. *Ann Rev. Entomol.* 27, 21–48. doi: 10.1146/annurev.en.27.010182.000321

Wikel, S. K. (1996). Host immunity to ticks. *Ann. Rev. Entomol.* 41, 1–22. doi: 10.1146/annurev.en.41.010196.000245

Wikel, S. K., and Whelen, A. C. (1986). Ixodid-host immune interaction. Identification and characterization of relevant antigens and tick-induced host immunosuppression. *Vet. Parasitol.* 20, 149–174. doi: 10.1016/0304-4017(86)90098-1

Willadsen, P. (1980). Immunity to ticks. *Adv. Parasitol.* 18, 293–311. doi: 10.1016/S0065-308X(08)60402-9

Willadsen, P. (2004). Anti-tick vaccines. *Parasitology* 129, S367–387. doi: 10.1017/S0031182003004657

Willadsen, P., and Kemp, D. H. (1988). Vaccination with 'concealed' antigens for tick control. *Parasitol. Today* 4, 196–198. doi: 10.1016/0169-4758(88)90084-1

Willadsen P. The molecular revolution in the development of vaccines against ectoparasites. *Vet Parasitol.* 2001;**101**(3-4):353–367. doi: 10.1016/S0304-4017(01)00560-X.

Willadsen P, Kemp DH. Vaccination with concealed antigens for tick control. *Parasitol Today.* 1988;**4**(7):196–1 98. doi: 10.1016/0169-4758(88)90084-1.

Willadsen P, McKenna RV, Riding GA. Isolation from the cattle tick, *Boophilus microplus*, of antigenic material capable of eliciting a protective immunological response in the bovine host. *Int J Parasitol.* 1988;**18**(2):183–189. doi: 10.1016/0020-7519(88)90059-8.

Yilmaz, B., Portugal, S., Tran, T. M., Gozzelino, R., Ramos, S., Gomes, J., et al. (2014). Gut microbiota elicits a protective immune response against malaria transmission. *Cell* 159, 1277–1289 doi: 10.1016/j.cell.2014.10.053

About the author

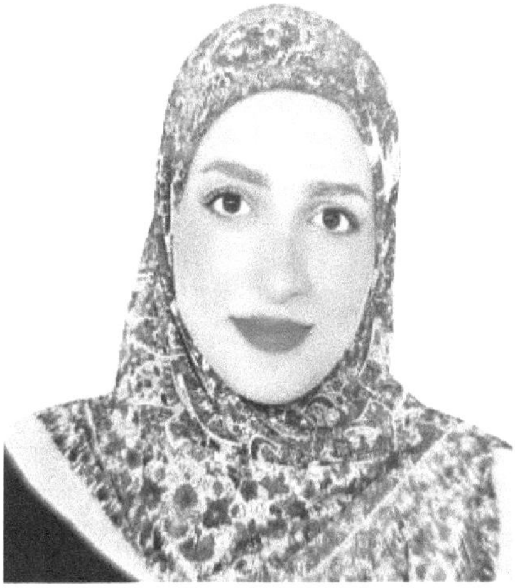

Dr. Mariam Kazim Jassab

Internal and Preventive Medicine

College of Veterinary Medicine Al-Qasim Green University, Iraq

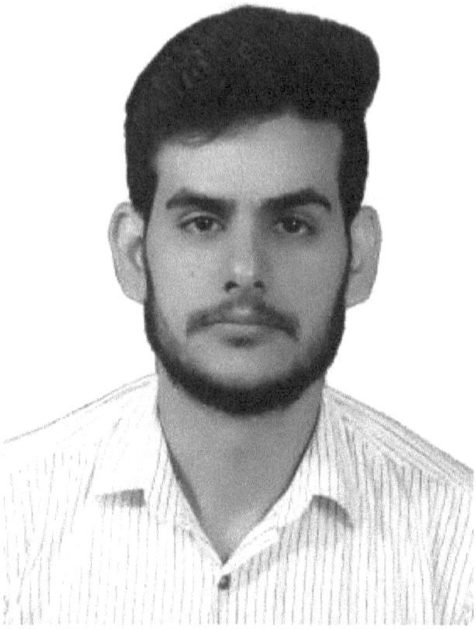

Dr. ALI ABOULKADHIM ABOULMAHDI

Babylon Veterinary Teaching Hospital, Iraq

FSC
www.fsc.org
MIX
Papier | Fördert gute Waldnutzung
FSC® C083411

Kolibri 360 GmbH
Ferdinand-Jühlke-Straße 7
99095 Erfurt, Deutschland
produktsicherheit@kolibri360.de

Druck:
CPI Druckdienstleistungen GmbH
im Auftrag der
Kolibri 360 GmbH
Ferdinand-Jühlke-Str. 7
99095 Erfurt